AF552858

ANIMAL MYSTERIES

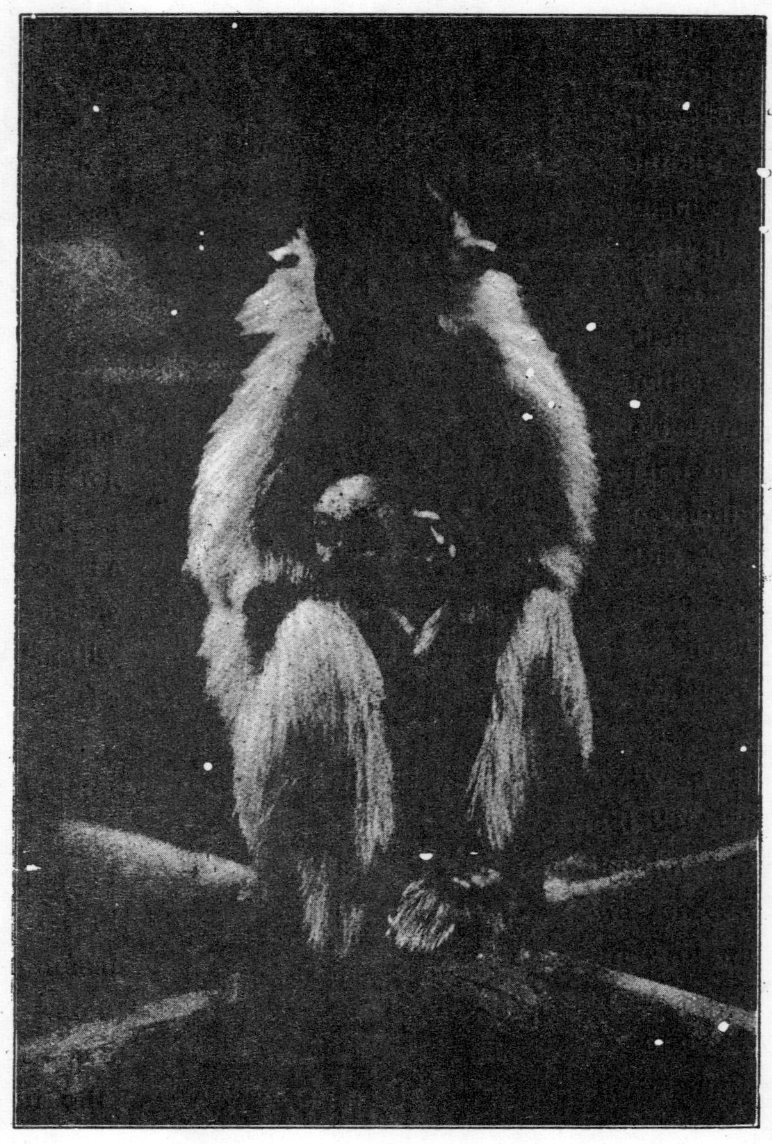

Sacred Langur Monkey with Young

Frontispiece]

ANIMAL MYSTERIES

By
E.G.BOULENGER
DIRECTOR OF THE ZOOLOGICAL SOCIETY'S AQUARIUM
ILLUSTRATED BY PHOTOGRAPHS AND DRAWINGS BY
L.R. BRIGHTWELL

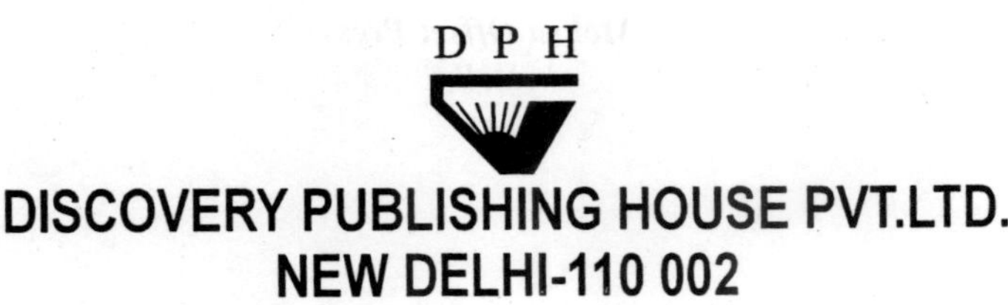

DISCOVERY PUBLISHING HOUSE PVT.LTD.
NEW DELHI-110 002

First Reprinted-1993
Reprinted-2011

ISBN 81-7141-226-2

Published by

DISCOVERY PUBLISHING HOUSE PVT. LTD.
4831/24, Ansari Road, Prahlad Street,
Darya Ganj, New Delhi-110002 (India)
Phone: 23279245 • Fax: 91-11-23253475
E-mail: dphbooks@rediffmail.com
dphtemp@indiatimes.com

Printed at:
Mehra Offset Press
Delhi

CONTENTS

LIST OF ILLUSTRATIONS

INTRODUCTION

In the Middle Ages man believed that swallows wintered at the bottom of ponds, that eels could be bred from horse-hair soaked in water, that newts "spat venom," and that toads carried priceless jewels in their heads. To-day of course we know better, and the normal schoolboy is better informed upon the ways of animals than was the savant of the sixteenth century. But Nature still presents us with a formidable array of unsolved mysteries, a few of which are touched upon in this volume. Teams of well-equipped scientists are grappling with the parts played by animals in our general economy,—their powers for good or evil. The migration of birds and food fishes, the laws of heredity as they affect our farm stock, the control of insect pests and germ-carrying animals,—these and many others are still very largely wrapped in mystery.

Glancing at those formidable tomes,—the catalogues of the British Museum of Natural History—the casual observer might well be excused for jumping to the conclusion that very few animals remain to be discovered. Yet every expedition brings back a host of species "new to science." One of the largest land animals—the Okapi—was brought to light less than thirty years ago. But still more enigmatic than the untracked forests is the sea, which for many years to come is likely to prove rich in the unsolved mysteries of the animal world.

If some of the chapters which deal with the habits and recreations of living members of the animal world, are entitled less than others to appear under the heading of "mysteries," it is the author's hope that they may for that reason not be found lacking in interest.

E. G. BOULENGER.

1927

CHAPTER I

SEA SERPENTS

AUGUST and September are months which herald that hardy annual, the sea serpent—nct in the flesh, but in the columns of the daily Press.

> " For the silly season is past and over,
> Gone with the equinoctial gales
> That sinuous hoax, the old sea rover,
> Curls the pride of his prancing scales,
> And the giant gooseberry misbegotten
> Lies in the limbo of all things rotten."

In recent years the topic may have been superseded by others, but from the numbers of letters that the writer receives from those wishing to ascertain his views on whether such a creature as a giant sea-serpent does or does not exist (the object being usually the settlement of a wager) interest in the problematical monster is obviously well maintained. The topic of the sea serpent is usually approached with diffidence, and received with derision or a flood of witticism. Rudyard Kipling's tale of the three reporters who actually saw the sea serpent, and had not the courage to "write it up"—save one who published his story as "fiction"—exactly epitomizes the popular attitude. The creature is often spoken of as though there could only be one individual in existence, a doubtless die-hard result of the ancient legends of world-wide circulation, concerning a marine serpent that lurking in some undiscovered abyss caused the storms and treacherous currents that take toll of the world's shipping. The possible existence of some huge sea snake is believed in by many naturalists of repute, whilst others would deny its existence even were they to see it exhibited alive in the Zoological Society's Aquarium. It is absurd, however, to dismiss the subject as a mere "silly-season stunt," for are not the strangest of beasts continually being brought to light? Less than thirty years ago rumours of an animal shaped like a giraffe and marked like a zebra living in the Ituri forest were not taken seriously. Yet to-day our national museum is the possessor of several examples of the okapi.

It must be admitted that all kinds and manner of things upon the sea-surface may very convincingly suggest a huge snake. Seals, turtles, schools of porpoises, masses of drift-weed, may all produce this illusion, and what could be more suggestive of a sea-serpent than the forty-foot club-tipped arm of a giant squid raised for a few moments above the waves. Such a spectacle presented at dusk and silhouetted against the sunset might easily convince the most blasé teetotaller on board.

As pointed out in a letter communicated many years ago to *Nature*, timber and masses of ribbon weed have been construed into a marine monster. To quote the writer :

"One morning I was standing amidst a small group of passengers on the deck of the ill-fated P. & O. s.s. *Rangoon* then steaming up the Straits of Malacca to Singapore. We were just within sight of the coast of Malacca when one of the party suddenly pointed out an object on the port bow, perhaps half a mile off, and drew from us the simultaneous exclamation of 'The sea serpent.' And there it was to the naked eye a genuine serpent, speeding through the sea, with its head raised on a slender curved neck, now almost buried in the water, and anon reared just above the surface. There was the mane, and there were the well-known undulating coils stretching yards behind. But for an opera glass, probably all our party on board the *Rangoon* would have been personal witnesses to the existence of a great sea serpent; but alas for romance!—one glance through the powerful lenses, and the reptile resolved itself into a bamboo, root upwards, anchored in some manner to the bottom—a 'snag' in fact—swayed up and down by the rapid current. A series of waves undulated beyond it bore on their crests dark coloured weeds or grass that had been caught up by the bamboo stem. Ignorance of the shallowness of the Straits so far from land, and the swiftness of the current, no doubt led us to our first hasty conclusion. But the story shows how prone the human mind is to accept the marvellous, and how careful we should be in forming judgements even on the evidence of our senses."

The reported appearance of the sea-serpent between the years 1520 and 1890 have been tabulated by a persevering Dutchman and his list totals about 250 cases. In the year 1830 one was observed in the Atlantic by the master and crew of an American schooner. Its neck was ornamented with a mane, and every time its head appeared above the surface it made a terrific noise similar to that of steam escaping under pressure from a boiler. In October, 1847, a specimen was observed off St. Helena by the captain and officers of Her Majesty's Ship *Dædalus.* The animal, estimated at over 100 feet in length, was described as having the head of a lizard with huge jaws full of long and jagged teeth. A few years later an account of a fight between a sea-serpent and a fishing party in Ballycotton Bay was described in the *Zoologist.* The monster on being shot at disappeared but not before disgorging a shoal of fish which when handled gave the most terrific electric shocks. In the same year a specimen was observed from a French man-of-war to struggle with and overpower a sperm whale. More convincing evidence of the existence of some huge serpent-shaped marine animal was given some years ago by the naturalist Mr. E. G. B. Meade-Waldo, a member of the Zoological Society's Council, and the late Mr. M. J. Nichol who was for many years assistant director of the Cairo Zoological Gardens. This sea-serpent was observed early one morning from the Earl of Crawford's yacht the *Valhalla* off the coast of Brazil. At first all that was observed was a dorsal fin about 4-ft. long standing out of the water. Below, the outline of the snake-like creature could be distinctly seen. Suddenly a neck about 6-ft. in length and supporting a turtle-shaped head appeared in front of the fin. For a very short period the animal moved in the direction of the ship at about eight knots an hour, but suddenly dived, and disappeared from sight for ever.

These modern sea-serpent stories are distinctly tame compared with those recounted by one Olaus Magnus, Archbishop of Upsala, who lived in the sixteenth century. According to this much respected dignitary of the Church, the Norwegian coast was the home of an enormous sea-serpent that snatched grazing sheep from the cliff-tops by way of an *hors d'œuvre* and would proceed to make a satisfying meal off a three-masted schooner with deck fittings, cargo and crew. His Grace professed to have been an eye-witness of these incidents which he not only set down in black and white, but illustrated with his own drawings.

The genuine sea-snakes of the "accepted" variety which swarm off the tropical coasts of Eastern Asia are entirely aquatic and extremely poisonous, a property which they possess in common with their not very distant terrestrial relations the cobras and coral snakes. Some fifty different kinds of sea-snakes are known, none of which measure more than six feet in length. They are all possessors of much flattened paddle-shaped tails which as a rule are prehensile, enabling the serpents to secure a firm hold by

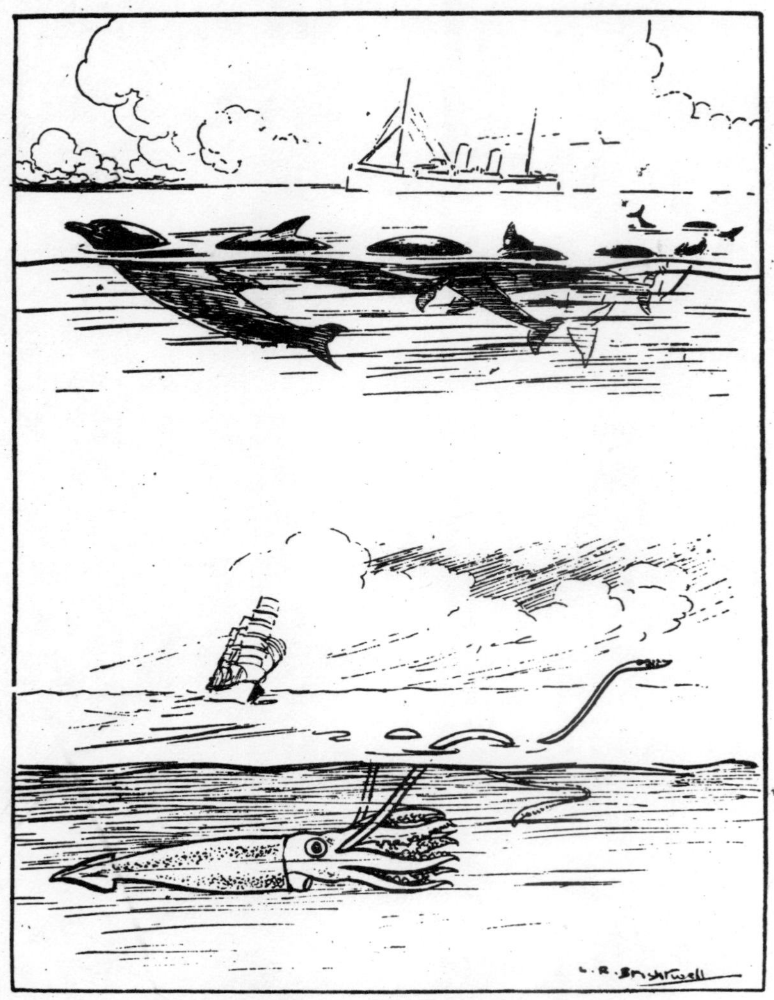

Possible "Sea Serpents"

twisting these organs round coral reefs, sea-weeds, and other objects.

Although they usually are found floating on the waves they can dive to great depths owing to the dilatability of their lungs which are capable of storing large reserves of air. The nostrils which are valvular and placed on the top of the head, are opened when inhaling air from the surface, and closed when under water. Their prey consists almost entirely of fish which are killed by the action of the poison before being swallowed. A deadly poisonous serpent having free range of the seas might well be regarded as invincible, but sea-snakes have many enemies.

Albatrosses and frigate birds fearlessly seize them and carrying them to some convenient crag or even mast-head, peck and beat them with their wings until they cease to protest, and pass away down the crops of the adventurous birds. Attempts to keep sea-snakes in captivity in northern climes have not been very encouraging. In the Madras aquarium, however, they do well, and share a tank with small sea-perches who appear to be on good terms with them. Prior to this the sea-snakes lived with the larger congers and dogfish but were hopelessly outclassed in the general scrimmage at feeding time. The small sea-perches actually seize food from amongst the reptiles' coils or even snatch morsels from between their jaws. The snakes suffer much from barnacles, but rid themselves periodically of the pests by moulting, when their "skins" are shed in one piece.

To return to the sea-serpent of rumour, fossil remains have doubtless played a large part in contributing to the general, if vague, belief in the existence of some gigantic snake as yet unknown to science. In the Fayum desert, for instance, recent expeditions have revealed vertebræ of a python that must have measured quite sixty feet in length. Pythons are largely aquatic serpents, and may be seen in estuaries so that the Fayum specimen when alive may well have caused some sensations amongst the possible primitive human onlookers.

Before now the vertebræ of a sixty-foot whale were presented to a trustful public as the last mortal remains of a veritable sea-serpent. Less than a hundred years ago a quasi-scientific charlatan—one Dr. Albert Koch—perambulated Europe with the skeleton of a monster which he called "Hydrarchus" or "The Watery King." When the box-office receipts began to fall off the doctor sold his 114-foot-long exhibit to the

Museum at Dresden, where the experts sorted the mass of bones. They found that the skull was that of an extinct whale, whilst the vertebræ had at one time or other been "worn" by five separate individuals of the same species. There was much excuse for the general credulity in those days when palæontology was only just born and was with difficulty struggling towards the light.

The sea-serpent may be explained away as being merely a strand of floating weed or a school of porpoises, as interpreted by a highly imaginative or even intoxicated traveller, but the more reasonably minded are willing to await further evidence and not hastily dismiss the creature merely because he has not been hooked. The fact that he has maintained a discreet silence up till now, does not preclude the possibility of his eventually turning up and confounding his critics.

CHAPTER II

ANIMALS—SACRED AND PROFANE

THE line of demarcation between religion and superstition is often very fine indeed. Animal emblems still revered by the Established Church have little or no significance East of Suez, whilst the elaborate tributes offered to many creatures in the Orient arouse the whole-hearted mirth of the respectable British church-goer. Rudyard Kipling has told us that we should thank God for not emulating certain Indian tribes and worshipping the crocodile. At the same time any man openly casting derision upon the sacred lamb depicted in all our churches renders himself liable to prosecution under the Blasphemy Act.

Many answers may be tendered to the question —What makes an animal sacred ? An impressive appearance has won many a beast immortal fame. The lion, the elephant, the eagle and the peacock, to name a few, have been revered on this ground alone. Again, an animal naturally associated with some auspicious natural phenomenon has been linked with the said phenomenon, and as a result won undying respect. The sacred ibis of Egypt has from time immemorial been associated with the annual rising of the Nile and the ensuing enrichment of the adjacent lands, whilst the dove's claim to religious and symbolic distinction is too well known to need elaboration.

Quite recently visitors to the Zoo had an opportunity of paying their respects to a notable example of a sacred animal—the white elephant. The beast was accorded a guard of honour from Siam to London, and once installed in Regent's Park was guarded night and day, and not allowed to be ridden. Until a few years ago the ceremonies attending the capture of a white elephant were most elaborate and impressive. The lucky discoverer of the sacred animal, were he the humblest inhabitant in the land, was raised to princely rank, paid a large sum down, and exempted from taxation for the rest of his life. The ropes used for securing normal elephants were replaced by stout cords of scarlet silk, and the animal was waited upon by princes and mandarins. Enormous feather fans were used by some high dignitary to keep insects off the sacred animal, whilst embroidered silk mosquito nets were employed at night. It was fed only out of gold dishes. In the early sixteenth century the natives of Pegu and

Siam engaged in a war which lasted many years —all over the possession of a white elephant, and in the course of the battles fought eight thousand men and five kings were killed.

Barnum, the famous showman, exhibited a white elephant in this country in 1883. Before receiving the animal his agents were made to sign an agreement embodying the following clause: "We have sworn before God that we will take the sacred elephant to love, honour and protect it from misery. If not we know the sin cannot escape hell."

The so-called white elephants are not white but flesh-coloured. The Zoo specimen appeared almost indecently naked, and some of the visitors' remarks on his personal appearance were hardly in keeping with the animal's sacred character.

The lamb, dove and eagle figure largely in our own churches, as does the cock—the emblem of St. Peter. Our public-houses and inns are often named after sacred beasts. This is natural enough since the inn is the direct descendant of the hostel which came into being for the shelter and refreshment of the pilgrims journeying to and from various shrines, notably in England that of Canterbury. Thus the "Lamb and Flag" of the Inner Temple is derived from the "Agnus Dei" of the Knights

Templars. The "Bull" inns refer to an episcopal seal, whilst Pelican and Unicorn signs commemorate creatures that received the Church's benediction in very early times.

The East although in some ways quick to acquire a veneer of "Westernism," still clings tenaciously to many old traditions. The elephant of India comports himself with a dignity consistent with the honour accorded him, and is represented in countless temples by Ganesh, the benevolent elephant-headed god of wisdom, happiness, and longevity. On the other hand the sacred bulls and monkeys of India amount to a public nuisance. The Brahmin bull, confident that none dare interfere, makes himself a disturbing influence in the public markets, whilst the sacred langur monkeys of the temple of Benares at one time became a regular plague.

The Brahmin bulls may be seen stalking along the narrow streets crowding the people right and left and sticking their ugly noses into baskets of grain and fruit without fear of being reprimanded. They become bold and insolent and do not hesitate to trample down whoever gets in their way. No one dare interfere and it would be safer for a Christian to kill ten natives than a single sacred bull.

The spoiled monkeys at one time did not confine their activities to playing "old Harry" in their temple, fouling the floors and destroying the vestments, but extended their unwelcome activities to the surrounding streets where no true believer dared prevent them stealing from the shops and snatching turbans from the heads of the passers-by. At last the British Government's aid was solicited to demand the deportation of the more intolerable specimens and a large number of these pampered pets were captured and sent to the Regent's Park menagerie where if the creatures were less revered their boisterous spirits and simian sense of humour were at any rate more appreciated.

In ancient Egypt the sacred baboon—the animal shown on the Monkey Hill at the Zoo—was probably accorded more honour than has been given to any other animal, before or since. Though at one time made to act as a professional pugilist, fruit gatherer and watch-dog, it was none the less deified and dedicated to Troth the scribe of the Gods. On ancient monuments these baboons are shown weighing the souls of the dead, duly recording the same and officiating at all kinds of dread functions. Hundreds of thousands of baboon mummies have been unearthed

at Thebes, each mummy set in the approved posture, seated bolt upright with hands placed upon the knees. In ancient Egypt the baboon coloured the people's life to such an extent that kings, priests, and court dignitaries wore upon state occasions imitation baboon tails.

Next to the baboon, the cat seems to have enjoyed most reverence—not only in Egypt, but also in Greece, and was exemplified in the cat-headed goddess Maflet.

Snakes are still worshipped in many parts of the world. Tennant has described how the natives of Ceylon in their religious abstinence from inflicting death on a snake are in the habit, when they have secured a particularly deadly specimen, of enclosing it in a basket woven of palm leaves, and setting it afloat on a river. The snake soon escapes and swims back to land.

The oven-bird of South America, which has a habit of plastering mud on its nest all day long is credited by the natives with a reverence for Sunday, and they affirm that on that day the creature refrains from all manner of work. According to Mr. A. Nicholls, "against the persistent assertions that the bird never works on the Sabbath it is vain to say that you have seen it bringing home and plastering mud on its nest without any regard to the Christian day of rest. The superstition sticks faster than the mud, and it will be further stated that the bird has only acquired its religious habit since the introduction of Christianity into South America."

As previously mentioned Rudyard Kipling alludes to crocodile worship. The species venerated is the " Mugger " or Marsh Crocodile of India and Ceylon, which is kept by the Hindoos in a state of semi-domestication. One of the most famous of the sacred crocodile ponds lies in an oasis north-west of Karachi. The pond is 300 yards in circumference and contains a number of little islands on which the crocodiles occasionally lie out and bask in the sun. The natives who worship in the neighbouring temples paint their foreheads red and have a special veneration for the largest crocodile, a monster fifteen feet long, to whom they salaam whenever he shows himself above water.

The Haje or Egyptian Cobra was regarded as the protecting deity of the world, but the honour bestowed upon it was as nothing compared with that accorded to the Scarab insect which has been represented in countless forms—from mural paintings and monuments to jewellery and royal seals. As all know the scarab lays its eggs in neatly fashioned balls of dung which it rolls along to its burrow between its fore-legs. The creature is always shown thus holding the precious sphere before it, and is regarded as an emblem of eternal life, the ball representing the earth.

The John Dory is regarded as an almost sacred fish in certain parts of the eastern Mediterranean where the fishermen liberate all specimens caught in their nets. It is often called St. Peter's fish, recalling the legend that this was the species from which St. Peter took tribute money, the two large circular spots, one on each side of its body, representing his finger marks.

That insect-hypocrite the Praying Mantis, so-called from the devout posture it assumes when resting on a shrub awaiting the approach of the small insects upon which it lives, is believed in many parts of the world to possess supernatural powers. It has a reputation for saintliness in Italy and Southern France, where the superstitious peasants deem it unlucky, if not a crime, to kill or injure one. An Arabian mantis is said always to pray with its face towards Mecca. The Hottentots actually worship the creature and, should a specimen happen to alight on one of their number, the lucky individual immediately becomes a saint. Even in Lutheran Holland there is something very like animal worship in the universal regard for the stork, and the bird which is represented as always bringing the babies is accorded state protection. The original cause of its adoration was due to its suppression of boring animals that once undermined the dykes. This is now abolished by the general use of concrete, but the good name which the bird once made for itself still persists, and the stork may be regarded as one of the few remaining sacred animals of Western Europe. The stork is unfortunately not as common as it used to be in Europe, and in Germany especially the number of occupied nests has greatly decreased in recent years. The reason for this is that the stork winters in South Africa where his food consists chiefly of locust and in the past few years the South African farmers have been waging war on the insect pest with arsenic. As a result it appears that the storks have died through eating arsenic-poisoned locusts.

The respectable rate-paying citizen who entertains such a contempt for the superstitions of the natives of various countries alien to his own, and who may even subscribe towards their conversion, makes quite a parade of establishing a black cat in his household—an animal that has ever been associated with witches and their like.

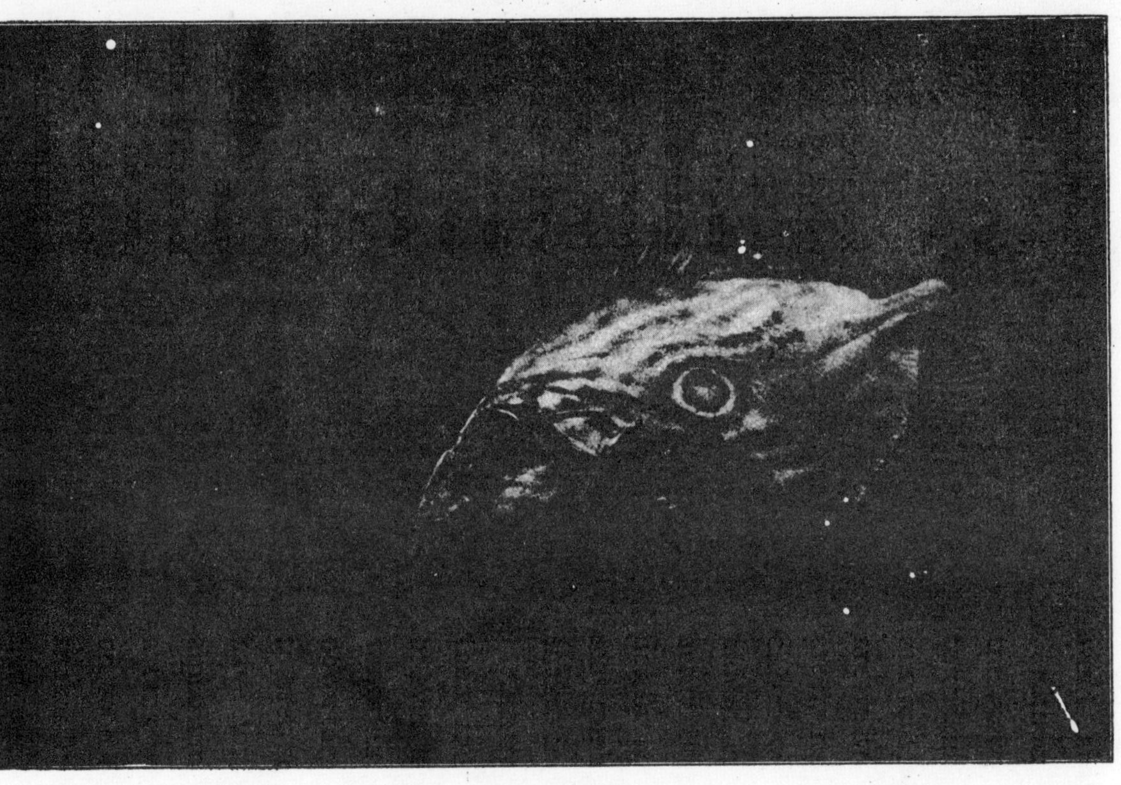

St. Peter's Fish.

[p. 30.

Man first paid homage to the black cat when many of the members of the human race were devil-worshippers. To-day in a civilized country the worship of the black cat still survives amongst a large section of the community.

Superstition is older than any of the established religions, and extraordinary survivals of it are to be met with on every hand. It dies very hard and makes a brave fight against education. This is specially noticeable in the less frequented districts, and aboard ship where men are cut off from their fellows for long periods. The Cornish fisherman for instance whilst afloat will never, for some obscure reason, mention the word "rabbit," and if forced to discuss the animal will make use of a subterfuge, referring to the creature as "they little brown things wi' white tails," or "You know, what Joe Tregenna shot the other afternoon." Similarly the northern trawlerman avoids using the word "pig" by substituting the term "grunter." The dread of reptiles and batrachians, inherent in so large a percentage of the world's population, is responsible for many strange superstitions. Anything with scales—bar a fish—appears to repel the average man, and frogs, toads, newts and salamanders, by reason of their peculiar movements and cold skins share in the reptilian anathema. Toads and newts are still accredited with the habit of "spitting fire," whilst the adder is capable of anything from sucking cows to swallowing its own young. Many a rustic who will cheerfully force into submission a vicious bull, quails before a crested newt, whilst the Madeira fisherman who, whilst not hesitating to tear the eighteen inch dagger from the tail of a giant sting-ray with his teeth, becomes almost hysterical upon seing anyone touch an ordinary wall lizard. On one occasion the writer whilst fishing off the coast of Madeira exhibited to his boatman a box containing a few of the olive green lizards which abound all over the island. The effect was electrical, and the fisherman was restrained with difficulty from throwing himself overboard. He would certainly have done so if the lizards had not been promptly committed to the ocean depths. The only reason the native gave for his behaviour was that the reptiles were evil, and that no good would come of meddling with such infernal objects.

The toad is undoubtedly the most useful of all Nature's night-walkers, and is the gardener's best friend. Yet annually thousands of toads are killed by ignorant rustics who in doing so believe that they are benefiting humanity. A toad superstition which is still given considerable credence is that connected with its supposed capacity for living incarcerated in solid rock for centuries. Experiments that have been conducted prove that a toad loses weight and vitality after thirteen months' confinement without food. Whilst specimens can fast for considerable periods, eventually like all other animals, they must take nourishment or die. The toads found walled up entered a chamber in the rock when very small—just after having transformed from the tadpole stage, through a fissure. They have survived and attained maturity in their prisons as a result of being visited from time to time by flies and other insects that gained an ingress through the same small fissure.

Another toad superstition—now almost dead—is that which has reference to the "toad stone" a supposed jewel lodged in the animal's head.

> Sweet are the uses of adversity
> Which like the toad, ugly and venomous,
> Wears yet a precious jewel in his head."
>
> *As you like it*, Act 2, Sc. I.

Old writers and the leading savants of their days had much to say on the subject of this stone. In the light of present-day knowledge, their writings are like one famous actor's description of a rival star's performance of Hamlet—" funny without being vulgar." All the old scientists agreed that "the stone may be found by exposing a dead toad to ants, and telling them to eat away the flesh." We have ourselves often conducted this experiment with a view to obtaining a complete skeleton of a toad, but somehow or other the "jewel" has always been missing. Toad-stones were affirmed to ensure one against various internal disorders, and were also believed to be a sure detective of poison. As the stone was apt to lose some of its virtue if taken from a dead specimen, it was recommended "to present the batrachian with a piece of scarlet flannel which would induce it to bring up the stone in its hysterical attempt to grab at the flannel." The three species of British newt are attributed with propensities similar to those once traditionally possessed by the toad. An allied batrachian, the Salamander, is credited with still more extravagant attributes. "Salamander" is a by-word expressing excessive heat, and is a trade term employed by a host of gas stoves, radiators, etc. Actually the salamander is a newt-like creature which does not like warmth, and in captivity to avoid its quickly becoming mummified must be kept in comparatively cool and damp surroundings. Pliny, the Munchausen amongst naturalists, sets forth that the salamander "is so intensely cold as to extinguish fires by its contact, in the same way as ice doth." Like the common toad the skin of the salamander secretes a poison harmless to man. The ancient Romans, however, believed its venom to be deadly and made a habit of dipping the live animals into cups of wine intended for inconvenient politicians. Needless to say many of their schemes went amiss. The idea of the salamander being incombustible took a long time to die. Even as late as 1789 the French Consul at Rhodes is recorded as having found one in his kitchen fire, and having secured it with the tongs. There are likewise stories of salamanders having been found in the craters of active volcanoes and one can only wonder how such beliefs originally arose.

In certain parts of Africa there is a belief that the hyena is the possessor of remarkable hypnotic powers. The natives state that it is capable of casting a spell over any solitary wayfarer, forcing him to follow the animal to its lair. It appears that the victim's only hope of salvation is to strike his head on the rocky entrance to the den with enough force to draw blood. This, so it is asserted, will break the spell immediately.

The goose barnacles that attach themselves by means of long stalks to floating timber from which they hang body downwards raking in food from the sea-water, were believed to turn into geese, a myth traced back to the 12th century and which arose from the desire of the priests to increase their limited range of Lenten fare by giving the birds a marine ancestry. They were said to grow on trees and to drop off into the water and hatch into geese under the influence of the sun's rays.

In many parts of the East attacks by leopards are regarded as avenging scourges. A black leopard is not looked upon at all in the same light as is a black cat in this country, and to meet one is believed by the natives of the Malay to be a manifestation of divine displeasure. The large monitor lizard is also unpopular. It is regarded as an evil beast and if one enters a house the owner in order to avert disaster employs a priest to go through an incantation. To hear the cry of deer is in many countries deemed most unlucky and in many parts of Eastern Asia to prevent the sounds reaching the ears of those attending a marriage ceremony gongs and drums are violently beaten.

A simple explanation for the tide is given in the Philippine Islands by the primitive inhabitants. It appears that in a far distant sea lives a gigantic crab who is very regular in all his

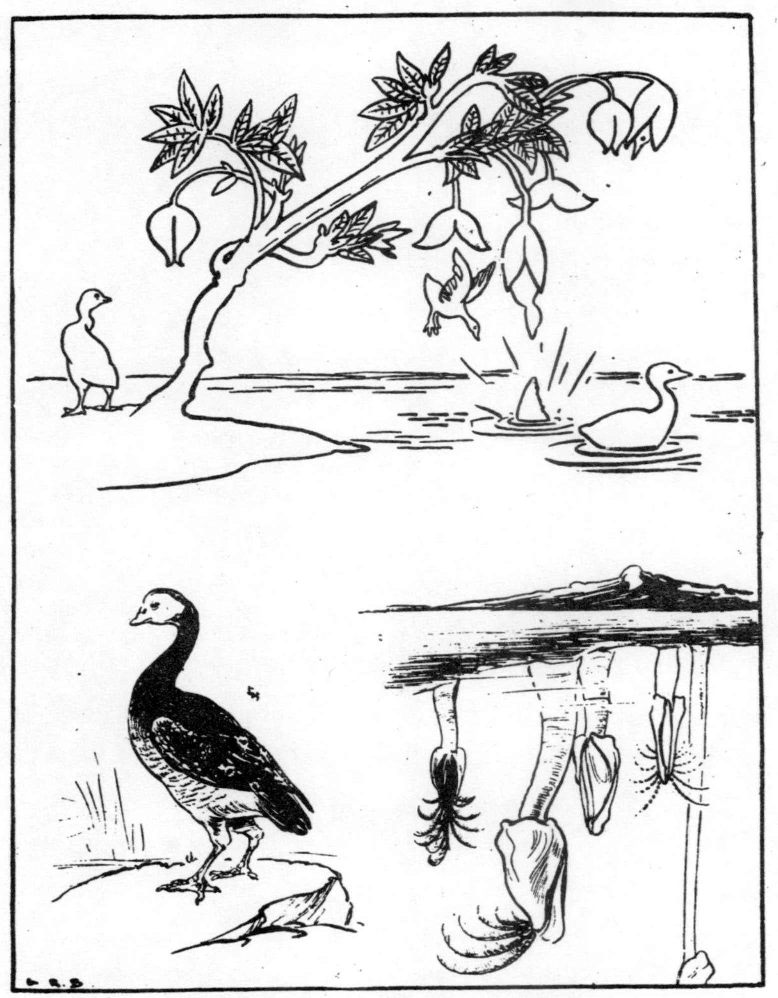

THE BARNACLE OF FICTION AND FACT

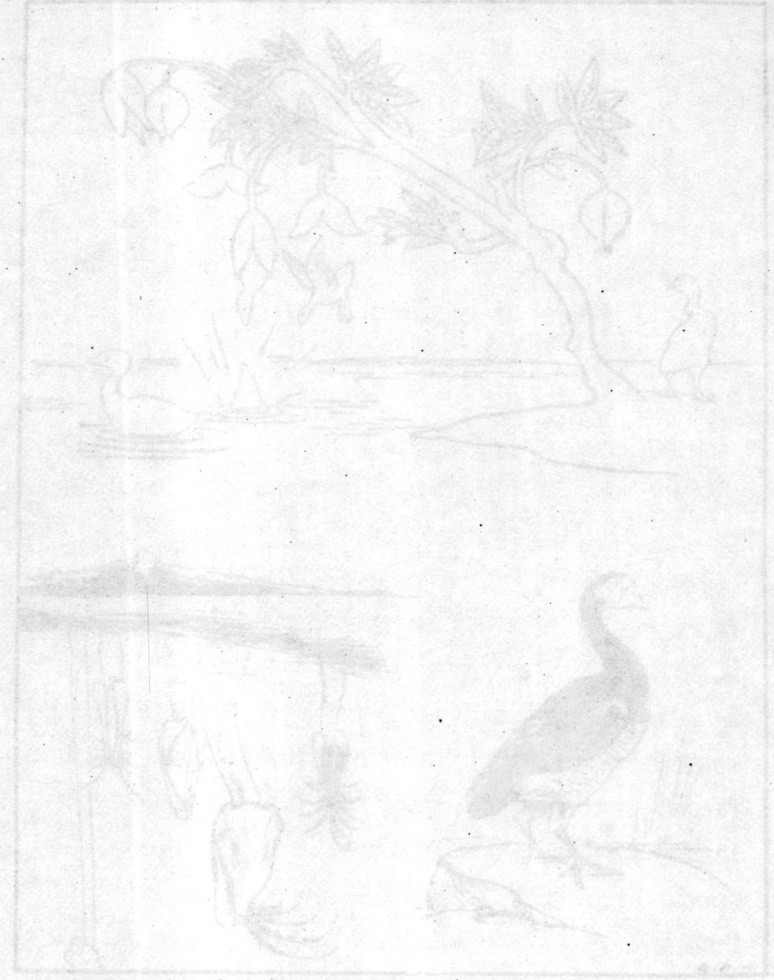

habits. When the crab goes into his hole, where he remains for twelve hours, the water is forced out, and accounts for the rising tide. When he comes out again the water fills up the hole and the tide recedes.

The horns of the rhino are regarded as exceedingly valuable by certain tribes of Arabs owing to the old superstition of their power to nullify any poison drunk out of them when converted into a cup. Hence, once a possessor of such a receptacle, one need have no fear of drinking with a stranger.

In the more uncivilized parts of the world the divines foretell events by means of good and evil birds. In Madagascar the kite is regarded as a creature of very ill omen and should its droppings fall upon the head of anyone that unlucky person is doomed to die. In the same country the laying by a fowl of an unusually large egg is ominous of something good, whilst an unusually small egg is feared as foreboding evil. No bird inspires more fear than the nocturnal Devil Bird of Ceylon,—a species of owl. Its cry has been described as a " shriek of torture followed by a gurgling sound as of a victim of strangulation." This unpleasant call being followed by a silence " as of death " naturally inspires great fear in the hearts of the superstitious natives. According to Mr. Gordon

Cumming the agonizing cry of the bird is accounted for by a gruesome legend in which a man having become mad with anger with his wife and child took the latter to a wood and murdered it. Then cutting off some of its flesh, he returned home and sending his wife out on an errand introduced the flesh into a curry she was preparing. As she was eating the curry the inhuman father told her what he had done. Crazy with horror the mother fled to the jungle where she committed suicide. In her transmigration her soul passed into the devil bird.

The Slow Loris of the Malay Archipelago possibly heads the list of mystery animals by reason of the unholy aura that surrounds it. Its supposed influence upon every place of human activity is quite amazing and often clashes with the British jurisdiction. For instance a native may excuse himself for having committed a murder by merely stating that a loris told him to do so. The animal may affect the harvest, kill by fever or cure of fever, make delay or annul a wedding and be responsible for any occurrence from a flood to an earthquake. The habits and appearance of the loris create an atmosphere of superstition in the minds of a simple and unsophisticated people. It has a grotesquely human shape, is

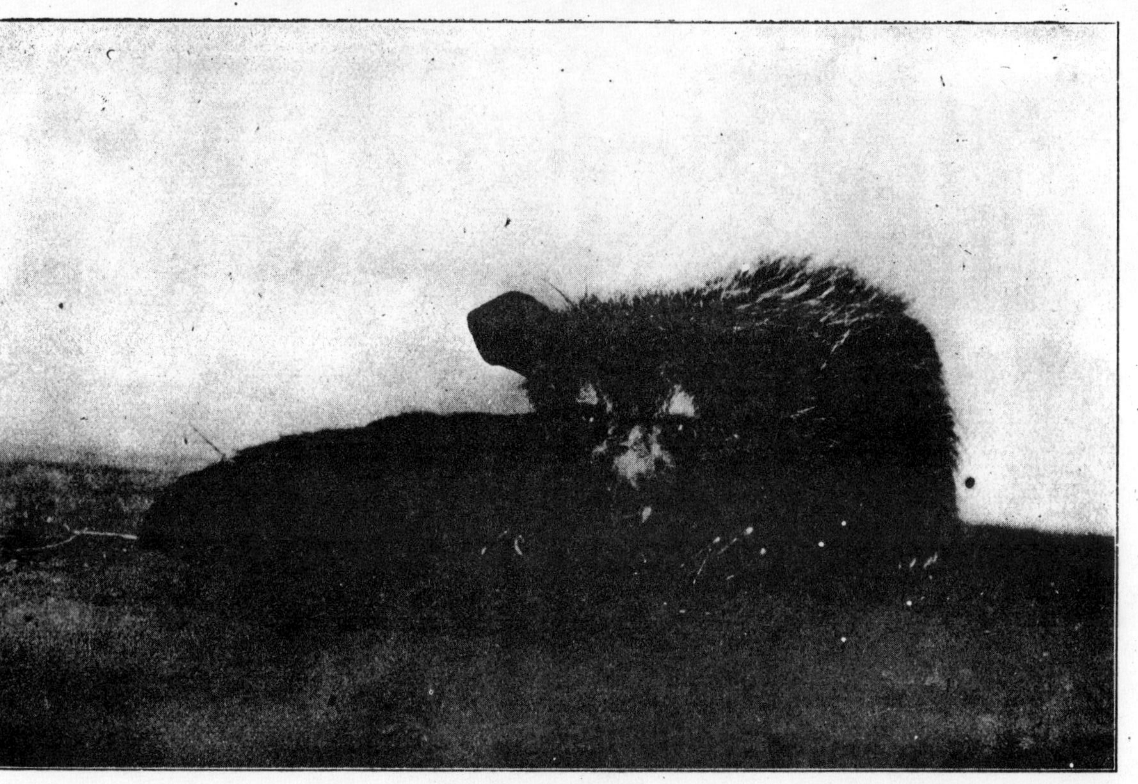

THE AYE-AYE.

[p.40.

deliberate—almost mesmeric—in its movements, and has enormous bulging eyes which it covers with its grotesque hands when exposed to light, a habit the Malays attribute to "seeing visions."

The Aye-Aye of Madagascar, an aberrant nocturnal monkey with a bear-shaped head and a fox-like tail, is another creature that is much dreaded in its native land where many strange rites were once practised in order to counteract its evil spell. The eyes of the animal like those of the Slow Loris are fashioned for seeing in the dark, whilst its great toe is extremely long and slender, and is used for extracting insects from the bark of trees.

To those whose passion for zoological investigation carries them beyond what may be observed in the Regent's Park menagerie the denizens of the realms of mythology and heraldry afford an interesting study. In the past theologians and philosophers, as well as anatomists, have disputed as to the nature, whether wholly human or wholly bestial, or a mixture of both, of the hipp-anthropoid Centaur and the man-faced lion, the Mantichor. The sages have also marvelled at the self-sacrificing Phœnix, a bird who finding that the heat of her body is insufficient to hatch her single egg, ingeniously sets fire to her nest and immolates it and herself in order that her race may be perpetuated. The Phœnix chick arises so fully-fledged from the ashes that careless observers have often rashly mistaken it for the mother bird, assuming that she had mysteriously renewed her youth by plunging into a bath of flames. The fiery destiny of the Phœnix is the more tragic in that she is denied the solace of a mate's company, there being no record of a cock bird, even before the egg is laid. Sad too was the fate of the Arabian Roc, which, as those familiar with the memoirs of Sinbad—that eminent mariner—will remember, was a bird of gigantic size and uneven temper. In spite of its enormous wing-spread it seems seldom to have flown far afield, and to this lack of energy and enterprise is due its present extinction, so lamented by ornithologists. It failed to survive owing to the disappearance from its native land of its only natural food, the elephant. The wanton destruction of the forests of Arabia, begun, alas, by King Solomon, deprived the elephants of the jungles from which they drew their nourishment, and their disappearance from that peninsula was accelerated by the voracity of the rocs which needed a whole elephant for a single meal. When the last emaciated pachyderm had vanished from what had become a treeless wilderness the rocs perished miserably of starvation.

The northern marshes of Arabia were once also the habitat of those remarkable creatures of which the sculptured portraits may be studied in the British Museum—the man-headed winged bulls, and the eagle-headed winged men. That an admiring humanity should have accorded divine honours to beings of so unusual appearance need not occasion surprise, but it is to be regretted that no record has been preserved of their dietetic preferences and that the excavations of numerous archæologists have failed to produce a specimen in order to set at rest the vexed question as to whether the structure of their bones was avian or mammalian. The same anatomical doubt exists about the nature of the famous Pegasus, or winged-horse, and the celebrated winged-lion domesticated by St. Mark. The winged Centaur gives rise to an even wider difference of zoological opinion which is only equalled by that caused by some of the creatures of Heraldry, such as the tricorporate lion, the three complete bodies of which dispute the possession of a common head, or the still more strange creature which is half lion and half ship. The Cretan Minotaur, human except for the head and shoulders which were those of a bull, had an ogreish reputation, the misbegotten freak, in spite of the graminivorous equipment of his bovine teeth and jaws, feeding exclusively on young maidens.

The appearance of the Harpies was calculated to shock the beholder as these poor girls had the legs and wings of birds and claws instead of hands. The winged Gorgons with their feathers and scales were likewise repulsive, their heads being covered not with hair but a mass of writhing snakes. Nor did their behaviour help to detract from the unfavourable impression caused by their unprepossessing appearance.

A Greek chronicler once asserted that the mountains of Cyprus were at the time of his visit infested by a nameless beast having the body and tail of a serpent, the hind-legs of a horse, the hump and neck of a camel, the fore-paws of a lion, the horns of an ox and the wattles and comb of a cock. Many may suppose this animal to have been the creature of only a more than usually exuberant Greek imagination, but the Hydra with its multitudinous and rapidly reproductive heads, and the inconvenient and almost jerry-built Chimera go far to match the Cyprist apparition in the multiplicity of their attributes.

But not even the griffon of which the cow alone

had wings while the bull was bald and spiky, can compete in popularity with that splendid creature of mystery--the Dragon. The devout find consolation in the fact that he is mentioned in Holy Writ, as indeed is his little cousin the Cockatrice, and it is only within quite recent times that the Chinese Emperors abandoned, together with their throne, the practice of ascending to heaven on a Dragon's back. It must be remarked that the Chinese variety differs from the English, Welsh and ecclesiastical in that his body is that of a sturgeon whilst his head is peculiarly his own. Also he is blue in colour. Amongst his Western kinsfolk whose paws are more bird-like, that colour is unknown in the best tradition, which favours white, black, red and green. A Dragon which is suffering defeat under the feet and sword of the Archangel Saint Michael has been depicted as having scales of so pronounced a character as to look almost like ruffled feathers. But although the Dragon usually relies for his protection upon crocodilian scales, still there is no absolute rule. Of the numerous species of Dragon described many had their bellies covered with a soft pinkish hide which offered inadequate protection to the lance of martial saint or errant knight.

The werwolves of the Carpathians, the werbears

of the Baltic shore, and the wertigers of Malaya were peculiar in that they assumed the heads of beasts at night only. Even more puzzling is the behaviour of the Transylvanian vampire which introduces meteorological complications by appearing at will as a fog, as well as in the shape of a man, rat, wolf or bat.

In the Highlands of Scotland otherwise blameless and respectable old ladies were wont to spend the long summer evening in the guise of hares, and naturally no one took the risk of annoying a creature that might happen to be one's own grandmother whose harmless seasonal indulgence had nothing in common with the sinister practice of the Continental vampires and werwolves.

Mermaids were quite a vogue in public aquaria and freak shows fifty years ago, and the old Westminster aquarium " featured " several talented ladies, who with nether portion encased in scales delighted the crowd with their beauty and fish-like grace beneath the water. One of these " mermaids " met with a somewhat unsettling experience. Amongst the lady's many unsuccessful suitors was a certain vindictive furnace-man whose duty it was to keep the water in the exhibition tank at an equable temperature. Smarting under his charmer's indifference he one day suddenly so raised the temperature of the tank that the performance came to a premature close, due to the sea-maiden splitting her fish-tail, and conveying to a convulsed audience in very unfairy-like language the fact that an attempt was being made to boil her alive.

Not long ago a "genuine" mermaid (stuffed) was on sale at an East End store. Examination by the writer, however, proved the mermaid to consist of a shameless blend of a shark's body and a monkey's head with certain embellishments that commended themselves to its "creator."

The classic mermaid is still popular with the poets and the painters, but most people, taking their cue from the scientists have ceased to regard her seriously. It was far otherwise at one time—even so late as the early eighteenth century. The sea still holds many secrets, but in the days before the dredge was known, it was credited with containing almost anything. Old-time naturalists and the illustrators of their works were prepared to invest all kinds of animals with human faces, and it is likely that the seal, sea-lion, porpoise, and especially the dugong or sea-cow all played their part in establishing a belief in the quasi-human inhabitants of the sea. Such writers as Pliny, Olaus Magnus, and later still the guileless Sir John de Mandeville revelled in mermen and mermaids, who were accredited with accompanying vessels for hundreds of miles. As late as the year 1663 a company of Dutch soldiers with their officers, bathing from the beach at Amboyna, saw a number of mermaids with long hair disporting themselves in the waves. Such stories might be quoted *ad lib.*, and one can but regret the camera had not been invented at an earlier date. Although such accounts are not to be taken seriously, they should at least command some respect, for mermaids were not only realities to the illiterate, but were actually seen and firmly believed in by many intellectuals both at home and abroad for thousands of years. What is the explanation? There is little doubt that the creature responsible for most of these stories was the dugong or manatee, a purely aquatic mammal which by reason of commercial rapacity is fast becoming extinct. The manatee yields a large supply of oil, its flesh is good to eat, and its skin can be utilized in many ways Nothing more could be needed in order to ensure its being hounded to death.

Naturalists are still at variance as to whether it is a sea-beast that is trying to fit itself for a life ashore or a land animal that has taken permanently to the water. All are agreed, however,

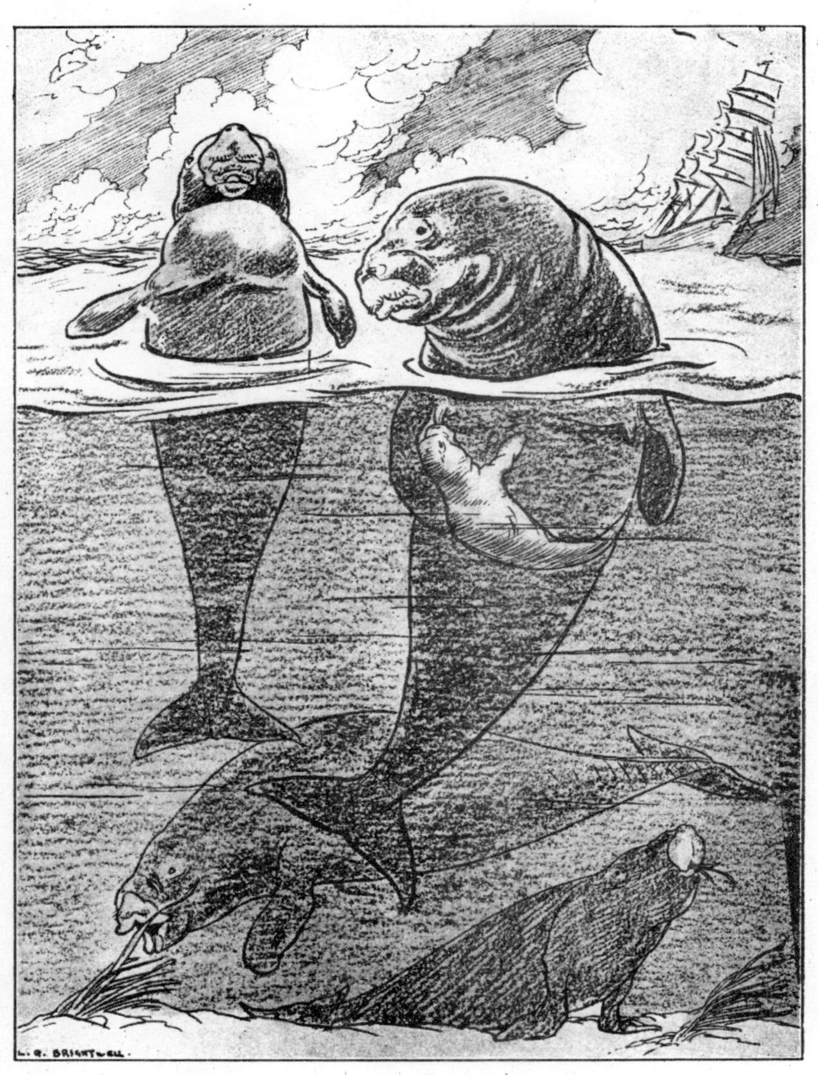

"MERMAIDS"—DUGONG.

f.p. 48.

that it is a near relative of the elephant, and fossil remains prove that at one time it had a much wider range than it now enjoys. It is a strict vegetarian feeding on the succulent weeds growing on the sea-bed or river bottom. The upper lip is split into two huge lobes or pads that pluck the weeds as might some giant finger and thumb. It is further lined with long bristles which act as sort of " soup strainers."

The sea-cows, scientifically known as the *Sirenia*, an echo of bygone beliefs, are grotesquely human-looking creatures, especially the large breasted females which are given to posing waist high out of the water, and one can therefore readily excuse the early sailormen for regarding them as almost human.

CHAPTER III

NIGHT LIGHTS

THE cause of almost every phenomenon can be explained, although it must be admitted that many matters capable of a perfectly natural explanation are apt to create in us a sense of mystery and "eeriness." Night lights are to be numbered amongst such phenomena. Even the most sophisticated is impressed with a slight sense of the uncanny when seeing the cold green of a cat's eye glowing in the dark, or when on board ship at night a fish darts from the bow, leaving behind it a trail of livid blue that fades as swiftly as the lurid streak in the wake of a meteor. Night lights can be very mysterious indeed and lose nothing of their wonder by explanation.

A great many "night lights" are the outcome of certain bacteria that give a bluish radiance capable of penetrating the gloom. Ordinary sea water, for instance, if corked up in a bottle may generate these bacteria, and a flask containing a "cult" when shaken in a dark room will give forth a greenish blaze sufficient to light up and make legible a column of a newspaper.

Fishermen are still as a rule very vague in their ideas of marine phosphorescence. In the West country, for instance, they believe it is caused by friction, and the water is said to " burn " or is spoken of as being dirty. They seldom attribute the light to living organisms.

In the case of certain mammals and birds which may on occasions be luminous, the luminosity is purely the outcome of bad table manners. A meal taken with more gusto than refinement is very apt to leave its mark upon the clothes, and in the case of fish-eating birds which may often be observed to be brilliantly illuminated at night, the mysterious light is entirely due to the phosphorus emanating from the putrefying offal which has become stuck to the plumage. A long-haired monkey inhabiting Central Africa is reported as being " lit up" (not in the American sense of the term), at night, and causing terror to the natives. The explanation is to be found in the nature of the monkey's food fragments that may linger in the creature's fur.

Most fish—dead as well as alive—are luminous in the dark. We all know the War-time story of the special constable who saw a mysterious light on the Scottish coast, and rushing to the scene of action—at low tide—found a cod that breathed its last at a fairly distant period of time. Such lights are of course the result of bacterial activity, but the lights seen on living fishes are derived from one of two other sources. The light may be merely due to sudden violent displacement of myriads of minute luminous bodies in the water itself, or it may be generated by certain special external organs—"photophores," on the actual fish. The latter is the case with those fish inhabiting the abysmal depths of the ocean. The lights which they carry act as lures to many other animals enjoying a sense of sight. Most of the deep-sea angler fish carry a luminous organ; a few fishes have enormous "head lights" situated on their craniums, whilst many have the lights arranged in rows along their sides, such fish resembling miniature liners with every port-hole ablaze.

A small sea shark which lives at a depth of over 1,500 fathoms has its lower surface only illuminated. It thus sheds a light on the ocean floor in a manner that must be specially useful to the ground feeder. In the case of some fish the lights can be screened or directed as required by flaps of skin which are controlled by special muscles and serve as shutters or blinds. A Pacific

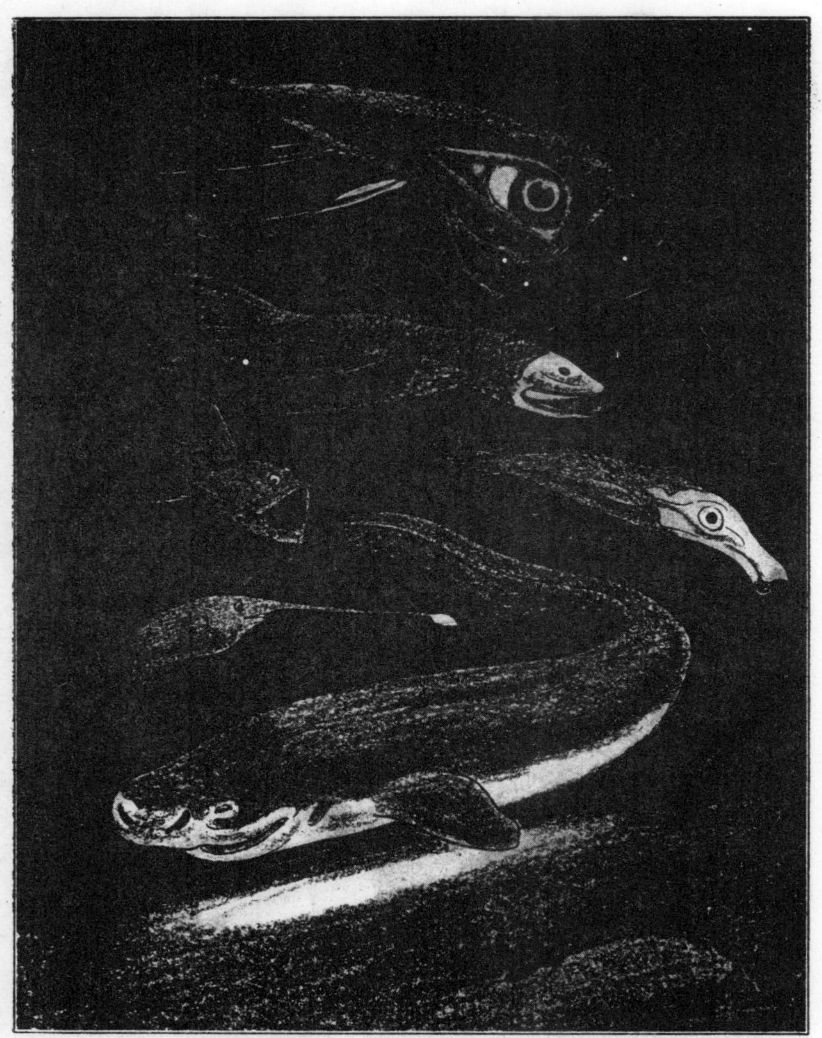

Luminous Fish.

[p. 52.

Ocean fish has two large light organs which burn by day and night, and these are cut out and used by the native fishermen who put them on their fish-hooks to serve as lures.

As already suggested these submarine lights help to illuminate the sea bed and to attract prey. They, however, also serve the purpose of the candles that ladies in the olden days set in their bower windows, for they are sometimes used in bringing the sexes together. The so-called glow-worm which is actually a beetle and not a worm, is a well-known example. Some genuine worms inhabiting deep water are highly phosphorescent during the breeding period when the males upon espying the brilliantly illuminated females at once gather round and fertilize the eggs which are expelled.

The sea swarms with luminous animals and the lights are worn in an infinity of ways. Some shrimps carry them at the ends of enormously exaggerated eye stalks; several large crabs have the abdomen only illuminated, whilst the Japanese marine fire-fly has light glands situated in the neighbourhood of the mouth parts.

The isolated patches of light seen on many animals are sufficiently impressive, but in the case of a deep sea prawn the light is puffed out ” in a series of smoke rings, the exact object of which is still obscure. The social squids of the Eastern Pacific are very brightly illuminated, the light not only attracting the prey but helping the members of the shoal to keep in touch.

Whilst most of these marine lights are of a green or bluish nature, lights of other colours are sometimes present. A squid living at a depth of over a mile has twenty-two light organs, two being ruby red, two sky blue, one ultramarine, and the remainder pale yellow. Another squid exudes its light in the form of rods of paste—like tooth paste from a tube—which are stored inside the animal and become brilliantly illuminated when they are expelled and come into contact with the water.

Insects appear to have been the earliest creatures to receive general attention as animal light bearers. Usually, as in the case of the glow-worm, the light which is disposed on the creature's under-surface is a " love light " attaining its maximum development in the perfect female, though observable in the pupa, larva and even the egg. The lady glow-worm is far more brilliant than her consort, and when out to kill coquettishly cocks her " tail " in the air to give the light beams a more extensive range.

Almost any organ is capable of developing a light produced by the burning of a substance called "luceferin" secreted in the protoplasm of the body cells, and which may be stored for future use. Thus a common New Zealand fly generates light in its kidneys.

Certain primitive insects that are found amongst manure and dead leaves are covered all over with light organs that flash intermittently. But from the spectacular point of view the West Indian fire-fly takes pride of place. Its green or orange light, described by Gilbert White as "amorous fire," has been turned to commercial use, and in Vera Cruz fire-fly farming is a regular trade. The insects are caught in vast numbers, being lured by means of small braziers into nets. Once caught they are stored in boxes, fed on sugar cane and twice daily sprayed with warm water. It is not difficult to guess the object of their capture. Night-life loving Vera Cruz demands huge numbers of fire-flies for decorative purposes. The insects are threaded alive on wires, and used to festoon garden paths and arbours, or are wound round the arms and waists of the local beauties.

The large fire-fly of Mexico was used during the conquest of that country, and we are told that the besieged army's overwrought nerves interpreted the light of the insects for the flashing of innumerable matchlocks.

The huge lantern " flies " of the tropics are enormous insects closely allied to the bed bug. They have hollow globes about the size and shape of a small finger, set upon the tops of their heads and these create a most powerful light. The larvæ which often assemble in large numbers secrete a dense waxy substance which in parts of Southern China is employed in the manufacture of candles. Some brilliant displays are provided by centipedes, one species abounding in chicory fields causing the whole area to glow at night, and the soil when dug comes to the surface in shining lumps.

Certain giant sea-squids—animals that multiply by the process known as " budding "—give out a very powerful light. When touched a phosphorescent light appears on the point of contact and Moseley has recorded the fact that he wrote his name with his finger on a giant four-foot-long specimen as it lay on deck in a tub at night, with the result that after a short interval his name came out in " letters of fire."

CHAPTER IV

WEATHER PROPHETS

THE elaborate apparatus at the command of the modern meteorologist ensures a fairly reliable forecast of the atmospheric conditions for some twenty-four hours in advance. The weather bureau is, however, a comparatively recent innovation, and at sea and in rural districts many still attach some importance to the signs and portents of the members of the animal world. In olden times man relied almost entirely upon the movements of animals to foretell the weather and in this respect many creatures, though frequently proving themselves very false prophets indeed, have gained considerable reputations.

Birds from the very earliest of times have been regarded as weather-wise. The swallow originally associated with all kinds of gods and goddesses is still regarded as a herald of Spring in northern climes. Frequently however the bird ushers in but a sorry travesty, its arrival really implying that in his winter quarters in Northern Africa the food supply is becoming less abundant. Similarly the bird's flight when persistently close to the water is regarded as a forecast of approaching rain, and this again is to be explained by an economic factor, a wet and heavy atmosphere causing the insect food to fly low. The swallow it must be confessed is but a poor weather prophet for, whilst setting forth from this country confident of a fair passage, it is frequently caught and killed by sudden tempests and even snowfalls. Some years ago thousands of swallows were thus caught on the French side of the Simplon Tunnel, and were saved by the humane railway authorities who loaded them into a goods train and released them in the sunshine of Italy at the far end of the tunnel.

Ducks often become extremely restless just before a thunderstorm. Their skulls are very thin and they are consequently extremely sensitive to sudden changes in the atmosphere. Hence a "dying duck in a thunderstorm" is a phenomenon by no means rare.

Donkeys are supposed to foretell heavy rain by braying loudly, a belief based on some substratum of fact, as male wild asses are known to call the herd together just before the advent of a cyclone or dust storm.

Many frogs, toads and fishes are famed as

weather prophets, not without some justification, in parts of Central Europe. The little bright green European Tree Frog is kept in glass jars provided with a ladder which it is supposed to ascend or descend, thus predicting changes in the atmospheric conditions. At the Zoo this method has not been found very reliable, although the frogs have been observed to become specially active and to advertise a coming storm by their croaking.

A small fish inhabiting certain stagnant ponds and brooks in Northern Europe and known as the Weather Fish or Thunder Fish, is supposed to prophesy the approach of bad weather. Some twenty-four hours before a storm these fish come to the surface and move about in an unusually energetic manner, a habit which has led to their being kept confined in small aquaria as barometers. In the case of this fish its restlessness is largely due to its air bladder being partially encased in a very sensitive bony capsule which conveys thermo-barometrical impressions to the so-called auditory nerves.

The voracious eel's excitability when a storm is at hand is due to another cause—suggestion. A thunderstorm usually means the partial washing away of the bankside, and the sweeping of worms, beetles, and other edible matter into mid-stream.

Hence a threatened storm arouses in the eel a joyful anticipation of an orgy, and in the fen district it was once common for fishermen to lure the fish from the mud by beating upon a drum, the eels always rising to the simulated thunder.

Spiders are said to be good at foretelling the weather. If it is likely to be stormy the threads supporting their webs become short. In anticipation of wet the creatures are very indolent, becoming active again when fair weather is indicated.

During his imprisonment at Utrecht, Quatremer Disjonval observed the relation between sudden changes in the weather and the habits of spiders. When the French invaded Holland in 1794 by crossing the frozen canals Disjonval looked forward to being released. An unexpected thaw however caused the French to consider a hasty retreat. But Disjonval's pet spider predicted an immediate return of frost, and the prisoner succeeded in some way or other in getting a message through to the French general. As forecasted the cold came again, the canals froze hard enough for the ice to bear the heavy artillery, and Utrecht was taken.

In the Regent's Park menagerie the wolves have earned a reputation for being able to forecast rain, their method of signifying a break in the weather taking the form of a prolonged chorus of discordant howls, repeated at frequent intervals for a day before the change takes place. Their predictions are almost invariably correct and the Zoo's head gardener can always rely on a period of wet weather when he hears this frenzied pandemonium.

The inhabitants of certain parts of Hampstead regard the sea-lions as weather-wise, having learned that when they can hear them barking rain is indicated. The barking, however, merely denotes a healthy appetite, and a reference to the Zoo's topographical position will explain the phenomenon —the sea-lions being only heard when the wind changes to the south-west !

CHAPTER V

ANIMALS AND MUSIC

THE love of music is a heritage handed down to all mankind since the first living thing arose capable of emitting sound, and it is indeed appreciated by many of those creatures which we are pleased to designate as the "lower animals." Before entering upon the part that music plays in the lives of birds and beasts in their native haunts, we offer the results of a musical experiment recently performed in the London Zoo. An orchestra consisting of two violins, an oboe, a flute and a mouth organ made a tour of the menagerie, visiting each house or enclosure in turn. The results were illuminating if somewhat confusing.

For instance, the rhinoceros was found to have no ear for music, and attempted to charge the orchestra, no matter what tune was played. The "Moonlight Sonata" and "Tea for Two" alike aroused his ire. The sea-lions on the other hand were delighted with everything put before them with the exception of "jazz." No matter how busy playing in their pond, they paused and rose to the surface as soon as the orchestra struck up. Most of the melodies that had exasperated the rhino delighted them, and they remained standing waist-high in the water until the last strains had died away. There could be no question of ulterior motives. The Zoo sea-lions always become elated when they see their keeper—associating him with fresh fish—but the orchestra offered no material reward for attention. Thunderstorms and war-time gunfire have no effect upon the sea-lions, so that mere noise cannot offer an explanation for their enthusiasm.

The Zoo's wolves and jackals responded all too readily to the music offered. A tune set in a minor key at once caused them to point their noses to the sky and give voice in so vociferous a manner as to drown completely the orchestra. The minor key, depressing at all times, had a like effect upon most of the animals. The cheetah thoroughly enjoyed "I want to be happy," but registered discontent and even alarm when favoured with Gounod's "Funeral March."

The orchestra when playing in the Reptile House never failed to bring the crocodiles to the surface. In fact every pond was emptied, the beasts clustering on the banks, and with heads upraised evincing the keenest interest in the performance. In the Insect House the like effect was obtained with the scorpions and certain spiders. All birds, strange to say, were in no way attracted. Some were obviously annoyed.

It is difficult to summarize the results of such experiments. Apparently one beast's music is another's discord, and what enthralls the emotional sea-lion exasperates the phlegmatic rhino. Animal songs that strike us as mere noises may tear the heart-strings of the creatures intended to hear them. The howl of the tom cat on the roof and the screech of the barn owl from the dead oak are equally approved by "specialized audiences." It is difficult to say exactly where "melody" begins and "noise" ends. In warm weather, for instance, millions of mosquitoes are done to death by coming into contact with the dynamos of our many power-stations. The "note" of the dynamo appeals to the males, and they flock to the danger zone, probably interpreting the engines' drone as a love-song of a possible bride. This failing on the part of the mosquito has been turned to account in some quarters. An American engineer has devised an ingenious electrical appliance giving out a particular note which attracts the mosquitoes in force, the insects hurling themselves

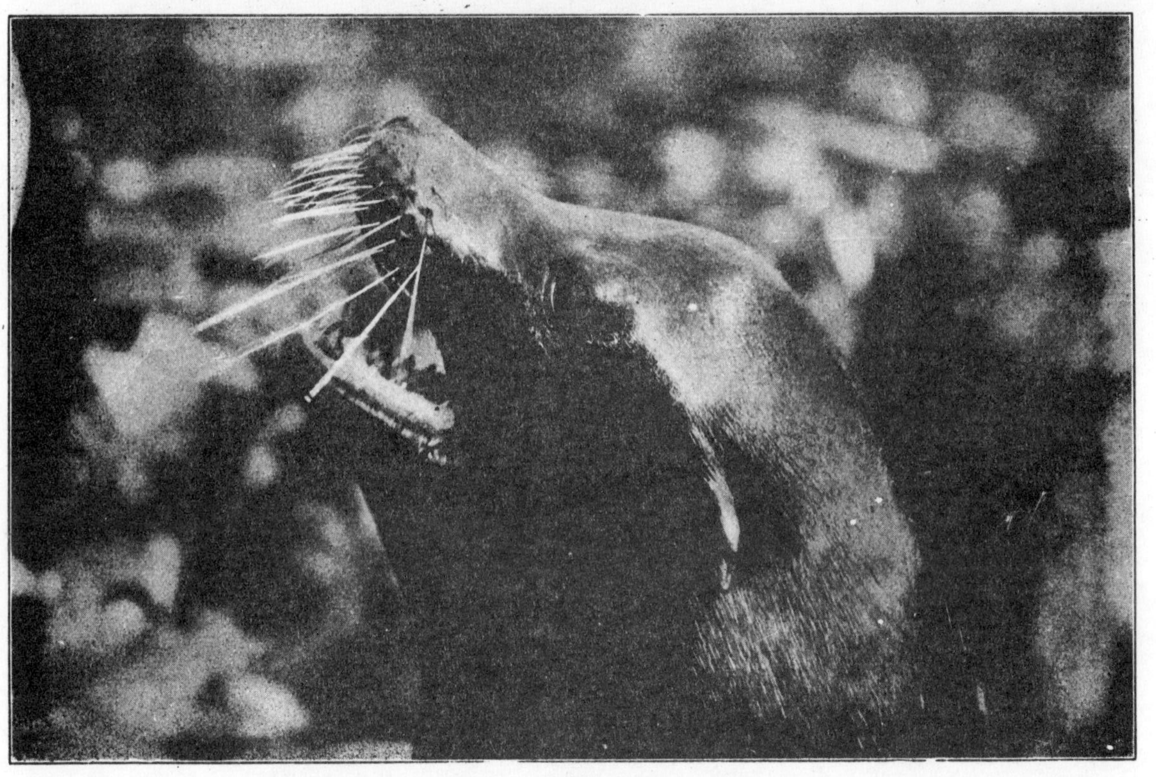

Sea Lion "Listening In."

[p. 64.

upon the apparatus, where they are at once electrocuted.

Spiders are said to appreciate music, and the sound of certain instruments will influence the creatures to come out of their hiding places and disport themselves on the floor or hang from the ceiling.

"I hailed thee, friendly spider, who hadst wove
Thy mazey net on yonder mouldering raft:
Would that the cleanle housemaid's foot had left
Thee tarrying here, nor took thy life away:
For thou, from out this seare old ceiling's cleft,
Came down each morn to hede my plaintiff lay:
Joying like me to heare sweet musick play,
Werwith I'd fein beguile the dull dark lingering day."

Anthologia Borealis et Australis.

Lutz who has written on the subject of spider lore recounts how the French author Pellisson when imprisoned in the Bastille fed a spider while his prison-companion played on a sort of bagpipe. The spider could be called to any part of the cell by playing on this instrument. There is an unhappy sequel to the story, for we are told that the governor of the prison learning that the prisoners derived entertainment asked for a demonstration. As soon as the music-loving spider appeared he crushed it under foot.

There can be no doubt that some animals are

fascinated by music, and such legends as that of Orpheus and the Pied Piper are based upon some substratum of fact. One myth enjoying world-wide belief dies very hard, i.e., the supposed fondness of serpents for music. No snake evinces the slightest interest in music of any kind. The dirge invariably played by "charmers" on their flutes is purely a piece of professional "bluff," the reptiles' dance being caused by the snakes fencing for an opening to strike as the charmer moves from side to side with a rhythmic motion.

Animal appreciation of human music is an uncertain quantity and not always flattering in its expression; but most animals enjoy the music of their own kinds—especially "love songs." Practically all birds become vocal during the mating season, but the Regent's Park menagerie can furnish other examples from very unexpected quarters. Many apes and monkeys have organ-like voices, whilst the alligators' oratorio and the frogs' choruses are other outstanding examples. The Siamang gibbon, the largest and most acrobatic member of the monkey tribe, is the possessor of an enormous throat pouch which can be inflated at will. It produces the most penetrating howls which on a quiet night can be heard at a distance of over a mile. The call of the so-called Howler, a simian inhabitant of the forests of tropical South America is likewise ear-splitting and the result of an over-developed larynx. One animal, the porcupine, lures his bride by rattling special sound-producing quills—a Romeo who woos his Juliet upon the castanets.

Only the male frogs and toads are endowed with a voice, the females being all but mute. In the case of many species the sounds produced are intensified by resonance in special vocal sacs, the throat being sometimes, as in the case of the common tree-frog, converted into a bladder-like pouch, which when fully blown out is as large as the animal's body. The voices of frogs and toads vary considerably. The croaking of the edible frog of Europe has been well rendered by the chorus of Aristophanes, βρεκεκεκεξ κοὰ κοὰξ. A tiny little South American toad gives a perfect imitation of the song of our British greenfinch, uttering a call which consists of a series of musical "rings," whilst a certain Brazilian frog is named "Ferreiro" or Smith owing to its voice resembling the regular beating of metal plates. Dr. Goeldi, of Para, states that "the ferreiro's voice is one of the most characteristic sounds to be heard in Brazil. Fancy the noise of a mallet slowly and regularly beaten upon a copper plate, and you will have a pretty good idea of the concert given generally by several individuals at the same time, and with slight variations in tone and intensity. When you approach the spot where the frog sits the sound ceases. But keep quite still and it will be resumed after a few minutes. You may discover the frog on a grass-stem, on a leaf of a low branch, or in the mud. Seize it quickly, for it is a most wonderful jumper, and it will utter a loud and shrill startling cry somewhat similar to that of a wounded cat." The North American bull frog is so called from the bellowing sounds which it emits when giving way to its emotions. The barking toad when annoyed utters a series of sharp barks like an irritable lap dog, but when making love changes the tone of its voice, the notes uttered during the breeding season resembles those of a powerful wind instrument.

The pretty little green European Tree Frog was some years ago let loose in the grounds of a large estate in the Isle of Wight, an experiment which caused its introducer, a naturalist-peer, considerable monetary loss. The frogs soon settled down, increased in numbers, and croaked loudly by night as well as by day to show their appreciation of their new surroundings. The little animals' efforts at community singing were, however, by no means popular with the human inhabitants of the neighbourhood, and when some years later the owner of the estate wished to sell he found that the value of his property had in consequence of the frogs' vocal efforts depreciated by several thousands of pounds.

Most frog choruses cease suddenly at the approach of a human audience, but they can usually be induced to resume their vocal efforts by an imitation of their croak.

Our capacity for appreciating music depends a good deal on the readiness of the performer to encore its own efforts. The incessant "music" of certain species of cicada can make night hideous, whilst the non-stop song of a South African cuckoo has earned for the singer the name of brain-fever bird. Insect music is not as popular in this country as it is in Japan, although Dickens's appreciation of the cricket's cheery chirp is echoed in many a country cottage. In Japan, however, the sounds produced by various crickets and grasshoppers, like those of the human performers of our concert platforms, have sometimes a market value. Tokyo has numerous markets where all classes flock to select their favourite insect musicians, just as our canary fanciers frequent the purlieus of Club Row and Petticoat Lane. In Japan the insects are housed in small cages of copper wire or bamboo which may assume the forms of temples, cradles, house-boats or lanterns. All classes are connoisseurs of insect music, and realize that whilst thousands of insects "singing" in chorus produce mere noise, a single chorister when isolated may be responsible for a simple yet beautiful melody. Each season has its special favourites. The cricket, herald of spring, comes first. Then follow the numerous grasshoppers and locusts, and finally the giant cicada, an insect two inches long with a four inch spread of wing. In the warmth of house or shop the insects may be persuaded to "oblige" well into the autumn. Before winter sets in the cages are thrown open, and the "artists" given their freedom—to hibernate, or lay their eggs and die before the first hard frost.

In modern Japan the picnic party may set out by car accompanied by a luncheon basket, and a cage containing an insect musician. In fact it is not an uncommon spectacle in the large cities to see a typical business man in quite faultless European costume setting out for his office with a neatly rolled umbrella, a severely practical despatch case, and an insect cage.

CHAPTER VI

FREAKS

A MISCARRIAGE of human law made by man for his own convenience and protection may have far-reaching results. Deviations on the part of Nature from her own laws, as yet imperfectly understood by ourselves, can likewise prove disastrous.

Ignoring some of the more repellent aspects of these vagaries, we shall concern ourselves with only those which may be considered of general interest and entertainment.

Very little is impossible when Nature blunders, and revolting and terrifying monsters are often the outcome. It says much for our improved standards of taste that the public exhibition of such freaks is on the decline: and only the medical and zoological professions may be said to be legitimately interested in such matters. The root cause of a freak lies in the embryo at the time when the component parts of the individual are in a state of flux. The result may be one upon which the healthy imagination does not care to dwell.

On the other hand a certain class of abnormality may be of the widest general interest since it casts light upon the ways and appearance of early forebears. That the young of most animals exhibit features reminiscent of their parents is a fact referred to in another chapter. The infant child and the elephant are both covered with hair at birth, the latter not only being as hairy as the mammoth, but having a short trunk similar to the trunks that must have been in vogue with its now fossil ancestors. Man may even come into the world with a tail which may persist throughout life. As a matter of fact we all possess a tail of sorts, an atrophied organ useless as a true tail. Its position and atrophy has much to do with our erect carriage. There are many instances of Nature leaping backwards many millions of years. Colts for instance, are frequently born with a complete hoof attached to each cannon bone. Primitive horses were three-toed and lived on swampy ground where the single toe of the modern horse would have been of little service. Shire horses are especially apt thus to revert to this bygone fashion, and although the extra hoofs are useless they suffer as a consequence no inconvenience or loss of efficiency.

The careful selection of abnormal animals and the steady development of such malformations has resulted in such useful "freaks" as the domestic horse and cow, and a formidable array of dogs, cats, guinea-pigs, rabbits, mice, etc. The only unfortunate feature of such scientific breeding is that the breeder does not always know when to stop. Fancy dogs, for instance, have in many instances, become so highly bred that their lives are made a burden to them. Ninety per cent. of bulldogs suffer from chronic bronchial disorders, whilst the champion skye terrier is at as great a disadvantage as the long-haired individual who used to be known to the showman as the dog-faced man. The hairless dogs of Central Africa, China, and Central and South America are the products of artificial selection. The dog is built much upon the lines of a greyhound, but attains a much smaller stature. It is entirely devoid of hair save for a tail tuft, and a clump of bristles on the forehead. Though the hairless skin, which feels like chamois leather, is not prepossessing, the dog itself is extraordinarily intelligent and affectionate. A remarkable feature is the degenerate nature of its teeth which are greatly reduced in size and number.

The pigeon fancy shows some still more regrettable instances of misdirected ingenuity, and no reasonable person can call the creatures surrounding the wild pigeon in our illustration " improvements " on the original stock. All must suffer much inconvenience due to the abnormal development of some particular feature. The " tumbler " cannot fly straight for more than a few yards, whilst some other " fancy " breeds cannot fly at all save in a dead calm. The more malleable an animal proves, the more it is "improved" upon. Hence the well-proportioned rock dove has been distorted into such by-paths as the Fantail, Owl, Satinette, Pouter, Punt, Trumpeter, Carrier, Dragon, Scanderoon, Short-faced Antwerp, Archangel, Barb, Satinette, Blandinette, Tumbler, etc.

Yet another freak of fashion is the waltzing mouse of Japan. Still popular in the Far East this breed is the outcome of systematically fostering a cerebral disease. The waltzing mouse is " born giddy." At any moment, in the middle of forty winks, or half-way through dinner, it may develop the dancing habit. It dances and dances round and round with ever-increasing velocity

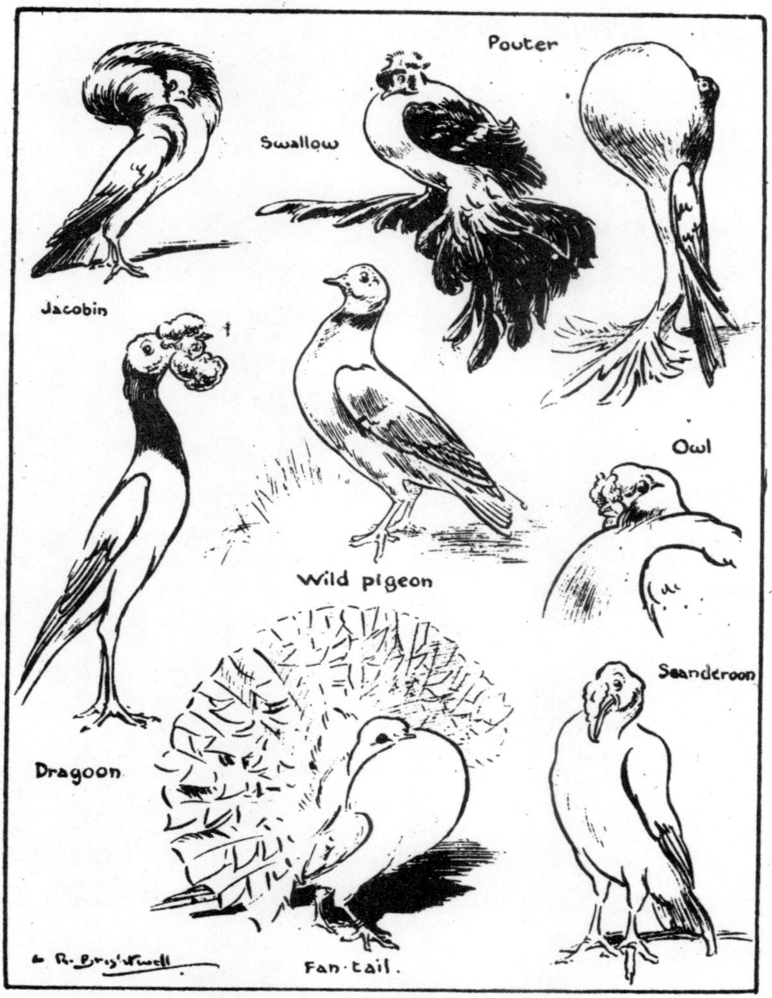

FANCY PIGEONS

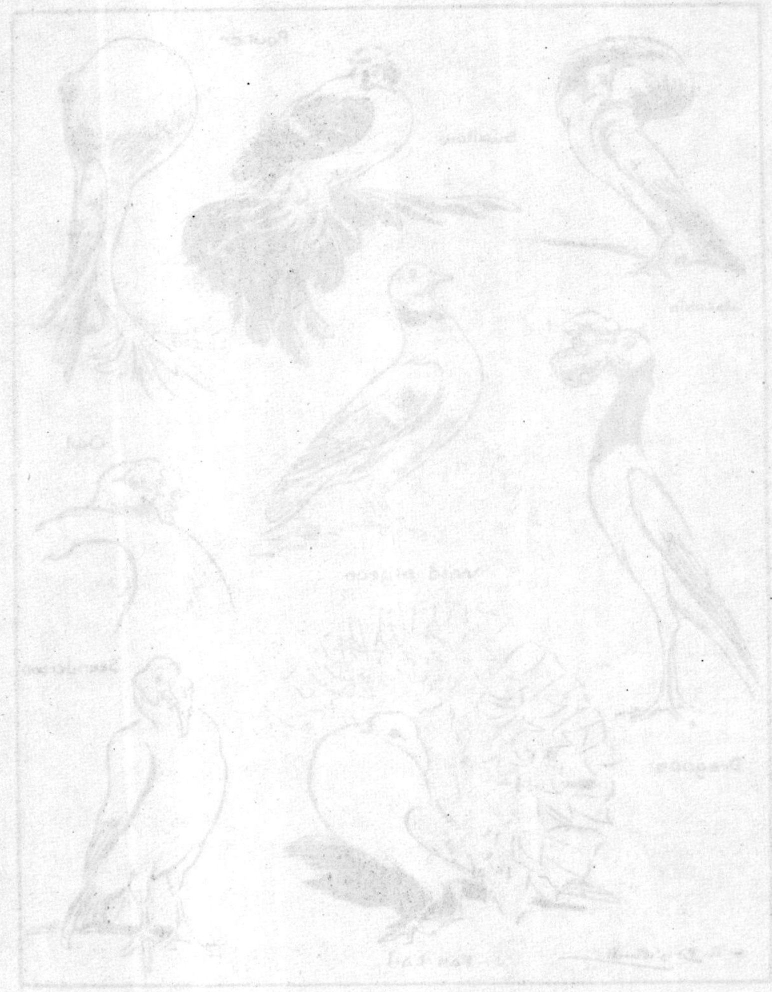

until it becomes a mere blur to the human eye. Then quite suddenly it stops and falls asleep again or continues its meal as though nothing were amiss.

A somewhat more pleasing freak is the long-tailed fowl, yet another creation of the Japanese. The bird is apparently a normal farmyard fowl, except as regards its tail coverts which may attain the amazing length of thirty feet. The birds are kept on perches in tall cylindrical cages. Once a day they are exercised on a spotless floor, the feathers being supported by a human train-bearer.

The Oriental's passion for greasy foods has led to the development of a breed of sheep in which the fattest portion of the animal—the tail—combines excessive adiposity with enormous length. In certain breeds this organ is so ponderous that the animal is provided with a small four-wheeled carriage in order to relieve the weight and prevent the tail from coming into contact with the ground.

The gold fish is another animal whose powers of adaptability have been abused, and a number of extraordinary varieties have been produced as a result of steadily developing certain exaggerations. A few are unable to swim properly, whilst one breed is doomed to perpetually turn somersaults. In the "telescope-eyed" fish and the "star-gazers" the eyes, which are enormous, project on slender outgrowths of the head. The lion-head is the latest ungainly type that has been evolved. It is perhaps the most grotesque form of all, as the top and sides of the fish's head are covered with thick growths, the latter bearing a supposed similarity to a lion's mane. The fish has to be kept in running or very well aerated water as owing to the thickness of the growth over the gill plates, the creature experiences a mechanical difficulty in breathing.

A fine specimen of the milk snake with two heads was recently found in the Bronx Zoo—an uncaged and unsuspected exhibit. Each head had a neck of two inches and was quite independent of the other. Sometimes both were ravenous at the same time, with the result that a card had to be placed between the heads at feeding-time, and care had to be exercised to prevent the food passage becoming chocked by a double stream of traffic. There can be no doubt that such an abnormality when discovered by the ancients sowed the seeds of such classical nightmares as Cerberus, Hydra, etc.

The old saying " two heads are better than one " is all very well in its way, but there is fortunately still a very healthy prejudice in favour of a single head per individual.

CHAPTER VII

NURSING FATHERS

WHERE there exists such an anomaly as a " nursing father " there is usually a " dancing mother " in the background. The human father who rocks the cradle, trundles the pram, or prepares a meal for a mother who is enjoying life at a bargain counter or the " pictures," has long been the butt of the humorist. But though, perhaps, envious at times of other more selfish men who make a bee-line for the club when the family becomes too vociferous, the nursing father may rest assured that he is not alone in his devotion, for in the animal world there are many instances of the male parent being alone responsible for the up-bringing of his offspring.

In the case of many animals both the father and the mother help to build the home, although the former, as a rule, makes himself scarce as soon as the family appears, which is not to be regretted, as the brutal male has cannibalistic tendencies and might be inclined to eat his young and make himself otherwise objectionable.

Amongst mammals the marmoset monkey is a charming exception. The male parent insists on enjoying the custody of the child, and takes sole charge of his son or daughter, handing the baby over to its mother only on occasions when a meal is due.

The feathered world offers several examples of the nursing father. In many birds both sexes share the task of nest-building and feeding the young. In the case of the rhea and the king penguin the burdens that fall on the shoulders of the male are exceptionally heavy. The rhea is one of the three surviving members of the ostrich persuasion, and is confined to the Argentine, where he is fast becoming extinct. Having won his bride by fighting for her with a rival wooer—a fight in which the long necks become intertwined in a serpentine fashion—the bird watches the disposal of the eggs, which are deposited in a communal nest. Should too many eggs be placed in one nest the males conveniently become broody, and any of the hens who seek to join the crowd of sitting cocks, and take a share in the nursing, are driven off with indescribable fury.

In the king penguin the father shares the nursing duties with his better half. The wife places the family eggs between her abdomen and insteps, and incubates them standing in a more or less upright position. When assailed by cramp or hunger she emits an ass-like bray, and her consort hastily shuffles to the scene of action. The two birds then proceed to stand shoulder to shoulder, the eggs resting on the lady's insteps. By a deft movement of her ankles she twitches the eggs on to those of her husband, and leaves him in charge until she feels disposed to return and resume her duties. Male birds which as a rule take no interest in the eggs laid by the lady of their choice have been known to make praiseworthy attempts to "come up to the scratch" in times of emergency. Thus some years ago a Japanese crane at the Zoo laid a couple of eggs in her enclosure which she sat on for exactly a month. At the end of that period a chick was hatched, and on its arrival the unhatched egg was ruthlessly turned out of the nest. Fortunately the male bird, who up to that time had taken not the slightest interest in the proceedings, immediately befathered the forsaken egg. He sat upon it for several days, and succeeded in hatching it, whilst the mother was devoting her entire energies to looking after her first-born.

In the sacred ibis, another bird which breeds in the Regent's Park menagerie, both parents take turns in sitting on the eggs, the period of incubation lasting about three weeks. The young are fed by both father and mother, the parents taking the bill of the young bird in their own and regurgitating half-digested food from their crops. During incubation it was observed that the father sat upon the eggs during the day and that the mother confined herself to night duty.

In a group of large birds known as mound-builders, the males raise enormous mounds of earth and decaying vegetable matter wherein the eggs are laid. The father is usually not only responsible for the building of the nest which may be over fifteen feet high and sixty feet in circumference but also for the welfare of the eggs. These birds have been observed at work in our Zoological Gardens. On being provided with abundance of suitable material the male parent seizes the leaves, earth, grass, etc., in his feet and throws them backwards towards a central spot. After a large conical heap has been formed and arranged to his liking, an excavation is made in the centre in which the eggs deposited are covered over and left to incubate.

Visitors to the Regent's Park reptile house in the spring are often attracted by the sight of a small toad carrying his eggs coiled round its [illegible] limbs. This toad is a native of Central and Western Europe, and is known by the name of the midwife toad, from the fact that its eggs, which are laid on land in a rosary-like string, and not in the water as in the case of the majority of frogs and toads, are taken care of by the father, who immediately they are deposited twines them round his hind limbs. The male parent carries his burden about with him for three or four weeks. He then makes for the nearest pond, where the fifty to sixty tadpoles that have developed within the egg bite their way through the tough egg string, and are liberated in the water.

One of the most remarkable modes of protecting its offspring is that employed by the male of a small Chilian frog, discovered by Darwin. The creature was at one time believed to be viviparous, but the fact has recently been revealed that the eggs—ten to twenty in number—are swallowed by the father as soon as they are deposited. The eggs develop within his large throat pouch, and the young frogs are retained inside him until they are able to fend for themselves.

By far the most numerous cases of nursing fathers are recorded from the watery world. The common stickleback is a splendid example. Having

Male Midwife Toad Carrying the Eggs.

[p. 84.

built an elaborate bird-like nest composed of reeds and twigs, he lures to it a succession of wives, which are wooed with an elaborate ritual. Each bride having deposited her eggs, the husband incubates them by violently fanning with his tail and fins—a task made the more arduous by the mothers' insistent attempts to eat their own offspring. The nursing father's solicitude does not cease until the young are hatched and some weeks old—when he dies, worn out by his parental cares.

The sea-horse, the fish which resembles the knight of the chessboard—well known to all visitors to the Zoo aquarium—adopts another method. The lady sea-horse lays her eggs in a special kangaroo-like pouch which is attached to the abdomen of the male during the breeding season. The receptacle is formed by overlapping folds of skin, and the babies when they emerge hover for a time round their father, anchoring themselves to his person by their long prehensile tails.

The male bowfin of the Great Lakes of North America makes a clearing among the rushes several feet across, and constructs a passage-way through the surrounding reeds, which he holds against all comers in a manner worthy of a

Horatius. He even guards the young for several weeks after they are hatched.

Finally, the little Chinese paradise fish may be mentioned as a perfect example of the nursing father. The male constructs a veritable fairy palace by blowing bubbles, made strong, adhesive, and resistive by means of a sticky secretion. He then proceeds to embark upon an arduous courtship, and his spouse, when won and wed, lays her eggs haphazard on the "floor," where they are collected by her indefatigable husband and placed in the bubbly nursery, where they eventually hatch.

It is possible, to judge at least from the jests and gibes of comic paper and revue—true indications of the mental trend of the people—that the respective functions of male and female among humanity will, in time, so overlap that the father will almost rank as a "nursing father." The advent of the female breadwinner, working in the City or going into Parliament, has made the pram-wheeling father a figure so commonplace that he is losing his ability even to evoke a smile.

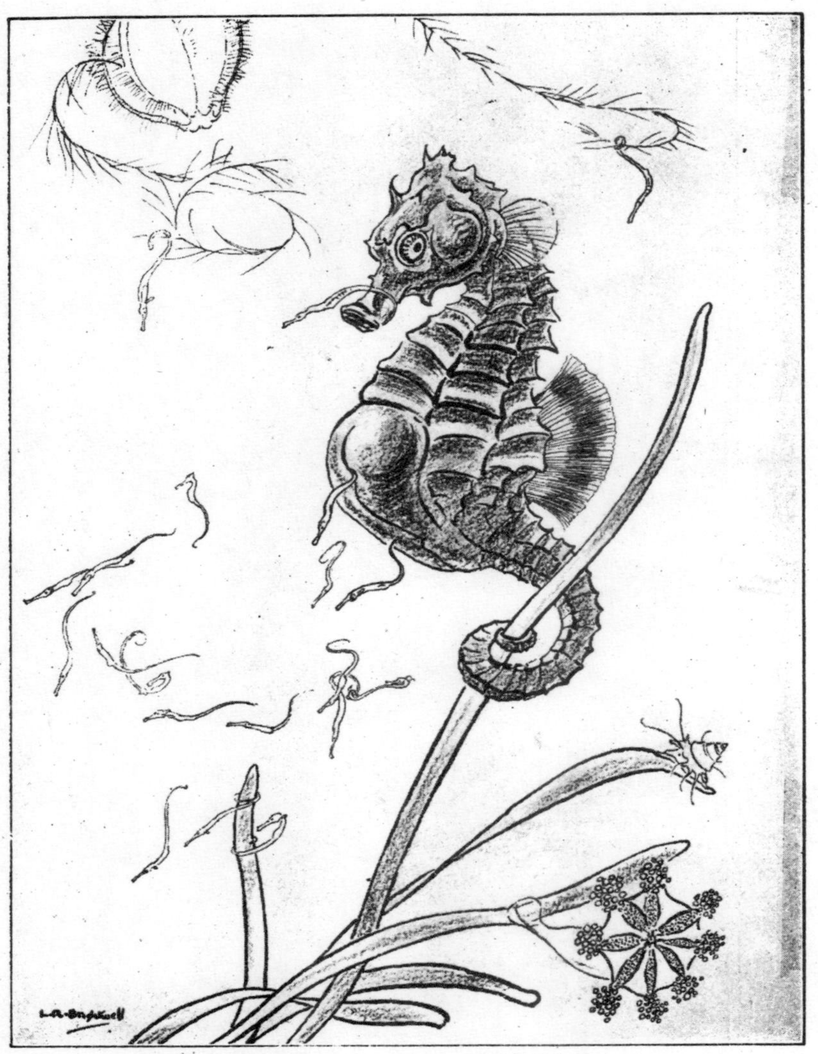

Male Sea-Horse—Releasing Young.

[*p.* 86.

CHAPTER VIII

EVOLUTION AS PORTRAYED AT THE ZOO

THE daring speculations which set the world by the ears in the middle of the last century are to-day part and parcel of the bedrock of our scientific knowledge, and are (except perhaps in Tennessee, U.S.A.) universally accepted. Few persons of education doubt that living plants and animals have attained their present forms only as the result of endless intermediary changes quite as dramatic—though more gradual—as those that cause a caterpillar to eventually assume the form of a butterfly. The study of embryology makes this still more evident, clearly demonstrating that the individual animal hurries through a series of widely contrasted forms, each more complex than its predecessor, before it is fit to face the outer world.

The study of evolution may not appeal to all as set forth in the text-book, but it may be traced in a more popular manner in the cages of the Zoo, where there are many witnesses to the slow but steady forward movement towards higher planes. In order to fully appreciate how first one and then another monster had its day before joining the great majority, a walk round the Zoo should be followed by a visit to the geological galleries of the Natural History Museum. At one period the invertebrates attained to immense proportions; later certain of the fishes developed a size and power seldom seen in present-day species, whilst at a later period—variously estimated at fifteen to twenty million years, the reptiles ruled the earth. The reptiles literally swarmed upon the earth, in the waters, and in the air. Some exceeded the whale in length, the giraffe in height, and the elephant in bulk. After the age of reptiles came a period dominated by birds. It is known that some far exceeded living forms, and were armed with teeth. With the disappearance of the toothed bird, the mammals came into their own. If we compare the fossil forms with the living it will be seen that modern birds, reptiles, fish and invertebrates are much smaller than their ancestors, but that mammals maintain a very fair standard of size. No prehistoric mammal exceeded the modern African elephant or the living cachalot whale in bulk, whilst if brain capacities are compared, the modern mammals are immeasurably the superior.

The fight for life has developed into a war of brains far more than one of tooth and claw. If mere armatures were the guarantee of success, the vast dinosaurs should still be encumbering the earth. The unrivalled collection of reptiles at the Zoo contains no creatures of large size—apart from the pythons, anacondas, and crocodiles, showing the reptilian brain's incapacity for expansion and development. The so-called giant dragon or monitor lizard of the Dutch East Indies is a dwarf compared to some of its ancestors, measuring but twelve feet in length, of which two-thirds is mere tail. Although a few birds appear to enjoy a greater æsthetic sense than the average mammal, their mental equality is much to be doubted, and their present high position in the scheme of things is largely due to the capacity shown by the majority for propagating their species in situations inaccessible to foes. The bulk of ground-building birds—from the partridge to the ostrich—only continue to enjoy existence because they benefit man. The ranks of extinct ground builders are legion.

At every turn the Zoo calls our attention to some creature whose ancestors have eventually found that certain ways of life suited their ideals, and every succeeding generation saw them more and more developed. Thus geology makes it possible to trace how the elephants by using their noses for browsing so fell in love with the idea that gradually their nasal appendages attained to sensational proportions. The giraffe's neck was not always the length it enjoys to-day, and there is little doubt that like the elephant's nose it has been stretched in a perpetual effort to attain to higher things.

Crocodiles and alligators have become admirably fitted for an aquatic life. When next at the Zoo ask the keeper of the Reptile House to remove a baby crocodile from its tank for examination. It will be observed that apart from possessing webbed feet and a compressed tail adapted for propulsion in the water, its eyes, nostrils and ears are all situated on the top of the head, enabling these parts to function when the animal is floating aimlessly about with only the head exposed. Further, it may be noted that the nostrils and ears are furnished with movable valves, which close when the reptile sinks below the surface, thus preventing the inflow of the water. The eyes in addition to a pair of eyelids are protected by transparent discs, whilst the tongue is so constructed that it forms a valve and prevents water from rushing down the throat when the mouth is opened.

Many other inhabitants of the Reptile House exhibit characters which in the course of time have become highly specialized. The gecko lizards and the tree frogs display modification of the toes which enable them to cling to smooth surfaces such as walls and even windows, whilst the arboreal chameleons, which are proverbial for the facility with which they change colour to suit their surroundings, have the finger and toes united in bundles to form grasping organs, and independent movable eyes, which turn in every direction.

A visit to the Aquarium will enable us to examine the sand-haunting flat-fishes, such as the sole, plaice, turbot, flounder, etc., in their natural surroundings, and appreciate the extraordinary changes which they undergo in the course of their infancy. Flat-fishes in their early stages resemble normal fishes, and swim in an upright position, and it is only when they are some months old that they take to a one-sided view of life. As the creatures develop they sink to the bottom, tilt over, and one eye, owing to changes in the formation of the skull, gradually turns over to the same side as its fellow. Thus is a flat-fish evolved, a creature perfectly adapted for a life in the sand of the ocean floor.

Many snakes have developed peculiar defensive characters. Thus the Hog-nosed Snake of America will sham death when surprised, the Cobras will sit up and attempt to intimidate the aggressor by dilating their necks, the expansion being produced by the distension of the skin supported by the anterior ribs, which are enlarged, whilst the rattlesnakes warn any approaching enemy of their presence by shaking their tails which terminate in the well-known sound-producing apparatus. Certain cobras have the power of spitting their poison, the noxious fluid being ejected to a distance of several feet and is always aimed at the face of the foe. This habit is most developed in the South African Ringhals, and at the Zoo when the door of the cage containing examples of this snake is opened, motor-goggles are always worn for the protection of the eyes. Why some snakes should have become endowed with a complicated poison apparatus, and others not, is a mystery. Originally snakes were all harmless, the poison gland of the venomous species being a simple modification of the normal salivary gland. That snakes are descended from a lizard-like ancestor is proved by the fact that certain kinds, such as the giant Boas and Pythons, are still in possession of rudimentary limbs, which are distinctly visible externally.

Some creatures are capable of producing electricity in their bodies, a phenomenon which may secure them immunity from foes and provide them with a means of attack. The electric eel of the Amazon River can transmit a shock which has been estimated at the equivalent of 400 volts. A very large specimen measuring eight feet in length living at the present time in the tropical hall of the Zoo Aquarium gave not long ago a demonstration of its electric powers, knocking clean off his feet a keeper who was in the act of cleaning out its tank.

Another peculiar instance of defensive adaptation is to be found in the small Horny Lizard of California, which confounds its tormentors by squirting fine jets of blood at them with tremendous force from the corner of the eyes, a habit no doubt developed by the reptile in order to interfere with the clearness of vision of its pursuing enemy.

The extraordinary anomaly of a mammal that lays eggs was for many years an unexplained mystery to the early settlers in Australia and the adjacent islands. Comparatively recently the

Monotremata have been assigned their true position in the scheme of things, and though they remain mammalian paradoxes, many of their affinities have been explained. Whilst having much in common with the marsupials, apart from laying eggs, they present a number of peculiar characteristics showing closer affinity to the birds and reptiles than do the ordinary pouch-bearing animals.

The Duck-billed Platypus, still fairly common in the neighbourhood of the rivers of Australia and Tasmania, has the jaws produced into a duck-like beak enclosed in a horny sheath, whilst a leathery flange of skin round the base of the bill acts as a sort of fencing guard and serves as a protection to the creature's eyes when it digs in mud or gravel for the snails and other creatures constituting its diet. A somewhat complex set of teeth is possessed by the young, but is shed before reaching maturity, and is replaced by a series of horny plates.

The animal excavates deep burrows by the water's edge in which it lives, and although largely nocturnal may be seen at all hours disporting itself in the water, often floating down stream on its back with the head and tail raised vertically. The mother duckbill has only a small pouch and

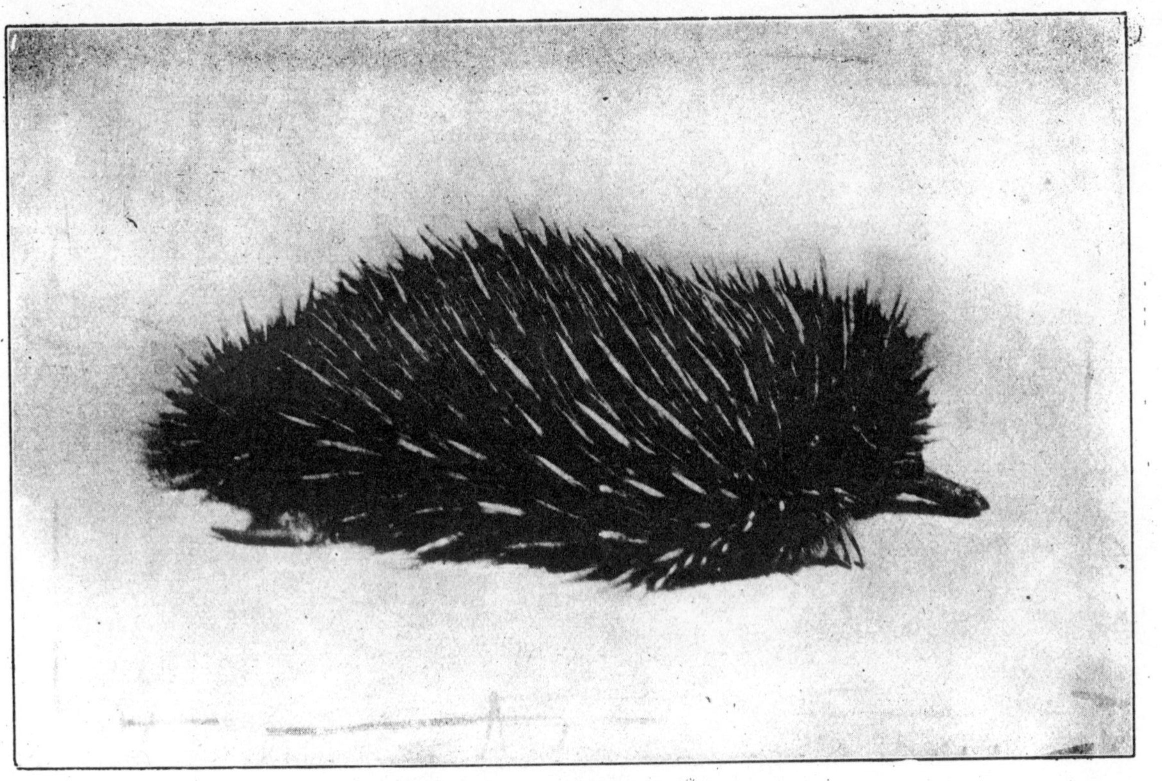

THE EGG-LAYING PORCUPINE ANT-EATER.

[*p.* 94.

her twin young, as soon as hatched from the very hen-like eggs, are held in position against the parent's body by means of her tail.

A strange feature of this peculiar creature is the so-called poison spurs which occur on the hind feet of the male. The spur is curved and hollow, and is connected with a gland which secretes a very poisonous fluid, and is used as a weapon for offence.

The Duckbill has lived for some months in a few of the Australian menageries and has survived a few days in the New York Zoo; it has never, however, been brought alive to England. Its cousins, the egg-laying Echidnas or Porcupine Ant-eaters, which enjoy a wider range, being found in New Guinea and Papua, in addition to Australia and Tasmania, are constant boarders in Regent's Park. The jaws of the creatures are produced into long bird-like beaks, whilst the entire body is clothed in a suit of sharp spikes. The strongly clawed feet are so placed as to give the creatures an almost deformed appearance, but they are nevertheless able to progress fairly quickly at a shuffling gait. When surprised or alarmed the echidna at once rolls itself into a ball thus causing the spines to stand erect and presenting to the enemy a very daunting appearance.

The steady if unconscious attempt upon the part of Nature to "better itself" is readily appreciated when one views some of the Zoo's "living fossils"—animals that have refused to move with the times, and having attained a certain standard of development have persisted in the same, whilst all round other creatures were preparing to meet a changing environment, or perishing as a result of their lack of adaptability. Several of these survivals from the past are housed in Regent's Park. The tapirs, one species of which is now confined to Malaya, and the other four to South America, once enjoyed a general distribution throughout the Northern Hemisphere. The survivors have altered little in general form from the giant tapirs that once roamed Europe. The practically wingless Kiwi of New Zealand—a descendant from a group of much larger flightless birds—is another ancient type. Its long bill with the nostrils set at the extreme tip is used for probing for worms. With its massive feet, which support its long legs and rounded body covered with coarse hair-like feathers, it is said to stamp on the ground, inducing worms to come to the surface, deluded into thinking that rain is falling. Some still more striking links with the past are to be found amongst the fishes.

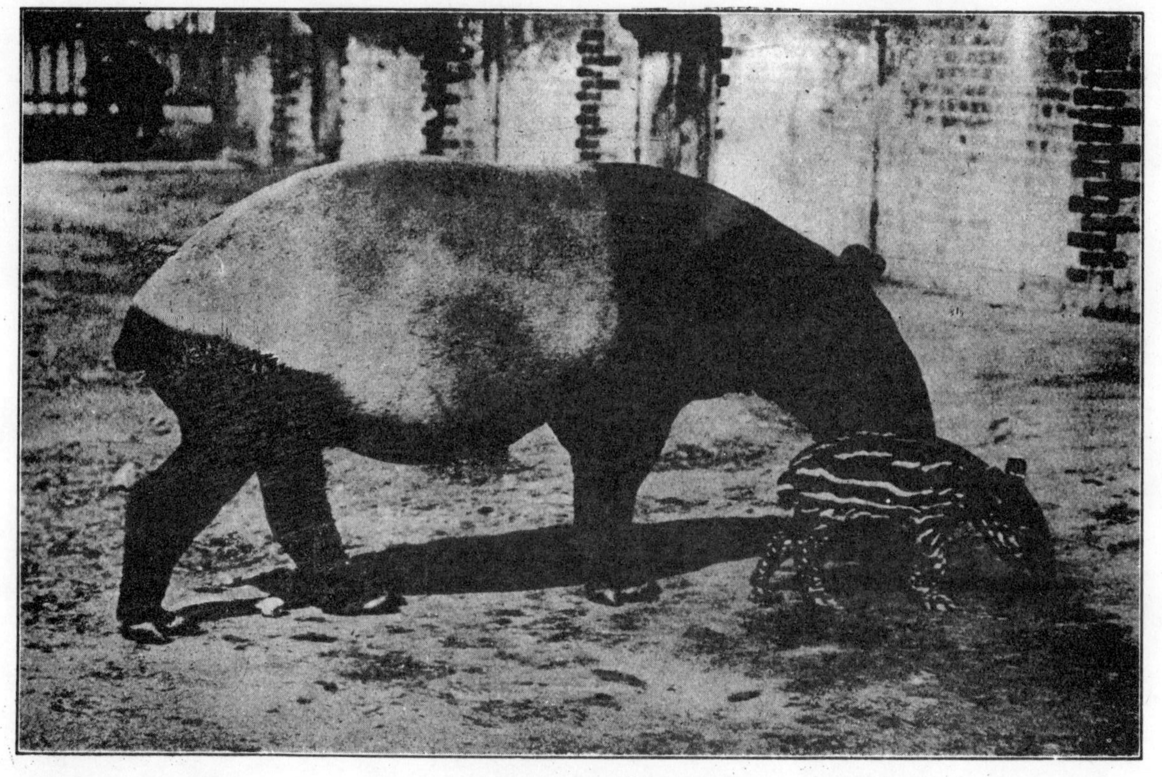

MALAY TAPIR AND YOUNG.

[p. 96.

Although the majority of fish are entirely aquatic in their habits and breathe the oxygen dissolved in the water through the agency of their gills, a certain number are able to live on land for considerable periods without suffering inconvenience. Some are even endowed with specially developed air-bladders which serve as lungs for the breathing of atmospheric air. A fish out of water is therefore not always in the deplorable condition that the popular expression would lead us to suppose.

Amongst those members of the fish tribe that are able to lead a contented existence on *terra firma* is a little fish known as the Jumping Fish or Mud Skipper, which frequents the river mouths of Africa, Asia and Northern Australia. Its muscular breast fins are developed into hand-like appendages which serve as the chief means of progression, these members supporting the fish and carrying it forward a distance of an inch or more at every step. Such a leisurely pace however would not be sufficient to enable the mud-skipper to evade the attack of an enemy, so when in danger it employs its tail as an additional means of locomotion. Curling the appendage forward and sideways it suddenly straightens it out with lightning rapidity, the manœuvre resulting in a leap of as much as four feet. The mud-skipper, whose large protruding eyes are situated very close together and like those of the chameleon can be moved independently and turned in all directions, spends much of its time reposing upon the branched roots of the mangrove trees. While thus engaged it leaves the tip of its tail immersed in the water, that porous member, well-supplied with blood vessels, acting as a respiratory organ for extracting the oxygen. At the approach of the dry season the fish buries itself under the mud of the river-bed, remaining below the surface until the rain once again fills the streams.

Quite as remarkable are the habits of the Climbing Perch found in India, Ceylon, Burma and the Malay Archipelago, for not only is this creature able to live for quite long periods out of water, but it has actually been observed in the act of climbing a palm tree, making its way up the trunk by means of its spiny fins and gill covers which are used as grappling irons. To prevent suffocation Nature has provided this fish with a peculiar receptacle on either side of the head for the storage of water. First cousins to the climbing perch are the Snake-headed Fish of Southern Asia. During the dry season when there is a danger of the water disappearing from the ponds and streams it inhabits it either buries itself in the mud or else migrates overland to fresh quarters, wriggling along with the aid of its long tail and fan-shaped fins in search of the ideal home. Snake-heads are often exhibited by the crafty Indian jugglers who, removing the fish from a tank and placing them upon the ground, force the creatures to promenade up and down in front of a mystified audience.

As previously mentioned certain fish are endowed with a double means of respiration, breathing with the aid of gills when in the water, but falling back upon their lung-like air-bladders when out of that element. During the dry season the Tropical African and South American lung-fish bury themselves in the mud making a cocoon-like nest wherein to repose whilst waiting for the returning rain to fill the streams and awaken them to normal activity. Whilst awaiting better days the fish breathe entirely by means of their lungs, receiving the necessary air supply through a tubular channel which pierces the roof of their temporary domain. The lung-fish exhibited in the Zoo Aquarium were all received in the dry state, and on arrival the square blocks of Africa or South America had to be broken up with a chisel and hammer in order to liberate the incarcerated animals.

Some years ago the address labels on a number of barrels containing specimens of a West African lung-fish destined for a private aquarium in Northamptonshire were found to be missing on their arrival at Liverpool, having become detached on the journey. The fish were therefore returned to their African port of embarkation where the barrels were re-addressed. Eventually they arrived at their new home in England, none the worse for having been out of water for over three months.

The natives are very fond of these fish, regarding them as a great delicacy to be eaten only on specially festive occasions. They dig them out of the ground and preserve them in dry storage until required. Several of these primitive fishes present external tadpole-like gills in their early stages. Even such comparatively "advanced" fish as the salmon and loach bear external gill-filaments, but they disappear very early in their owner's career.

The Tuatera of New Zealand is another "living fossil." At first glance it looks like a fairly normal lizard, but its affinity to the lizard tribe is only superficial, for actually it has more in common with living tortoises and crocodiles. It is the sole survivor of a group of reptiles—the Rhyncocephalia—which flourished before the dinosaurs arrived at their "lost world" state of inflation. A strange feature of the creature is its possession of a vestigial structure situated on the top of its head and which was once upon a time a third and functional eye. Being of a harmless nature and good eating it would long ago have ceased to exist, but for the Government protection which it enjoys.

In the Aquarium is a link from the yet remoter past. This is the King Crab, a strange creature also the possessor of a third eye, and one that has survived from a time when the dominant types of life were invertebrates. The King Crabs are closely akin to the trilobites—an extinct group of animals that once flourished in almost every sea. The creature's successful bid for immortality is due to its armour and the fact that it is of no conceivable use to man.

One of the most interesting phases of the whole study of evolution is the tendency shown by young animals to resemble their remote ancestors. Human infants for instance often make their debut in quite a thick coat of hair, whilst their feet show much of the plasticity common to those of their poor relations—the monkeys. The elephant comes into the world as hairy as the mammoth ; whilst lions, young deer, pigs, tapirs, enjoy spotted birthday suits, which they lose upon approaching maturity. The plumage of most young birds differs in a marked degree from that of the adult, and is often retained until its wearer has fully reached the parental size. The Hoatzin of South America carries the tendency to emulate its ancestors beyond mere coloration. Each wing in early life bears two well-developed clawed fingers, by means of which the young birds clamber about the trees. Although classed generally with the rails, the Hoatzin at once conjures visions of those strange birds that enjoyed life towards the close of the Reptile Age. Completely adapted to enjoy their divers ways of life as are many of the inhabitants of the Regent's Park menagerie, it is scarcely conceivable that they, or ourselves for that matter, have arrived at the highest pinnacle of development. Modern civilized man—despite what the pessimist may say is from the intellectual point of view as great an improvement on his forebears as is the living elephant on his rabbit-like ancestor, the hyrax, or cony of the Bible.

CHAPTER IX

UNINVITED GUESTS

A CERTAIN amount of publicity has recently been accorded to that bugbear of society, the uninvited guest. No social function is free from the nuisance, and the host smarting beneath such an affliction may perhaps find some consolation in glancing at a few fellow sufferers in the animal world.

A good example of a creature entertaining uninvited guests is that of the Prairie Marmot of Central America whose burrow is habitually invaded by the little desert owl and the rattlesnake. Old writers painted a beautiful picture of beast, bird and reptile living together in a state of Utopian harmony. Such a picture does not, however, quite square with facts, for both owl and snake devour one another's young as well as the newly-born offspring of the marmot, who being a strict vegetarian gets no compensation.

An instance of a more peaceful association is afforded by the New Zealand Tuatera Lizard in whose burrows live various species of petrels. The deep burrows which are invariably excavated by the lizard end in a divided chamber, and it has been observed that the tuatera always occupies the right side and the birds the left. Whilst tolerant of the petrels and their chicks, the tuatera does not allow any other reptile of its own kind to live in the same hole.

An uninvited but useful guest is the so-called Rhinoceros bird, a species of starling, which gathers in force on the tick-infested back of the large pachyderm. On the approach of danger the flock rises with loud cries, thus giving timely warning to a monster not blessed with a very keen eyesight. Also uninvited but not unwelcome to the host is the Spur-winged Lapwing, a bird that wanders fearlessly in and out of the open mouths of giant crocodiles, relieving the great reptiles of innumerable parasites. The crocodile has on more than a single occasion been observed to actually close its mouth during one of these visits and after a short interval to open it again to let his guest depart.

The vividly striped Pilot Fish has earned an undeserved reputation for being an efficient submarine guide, and extravagant stories are told by sailors of huge sharks carrying the smaller fish in their mouths and letting them out in order to investigate any suspicious object such as a net or ship's keel. Actually the active pilot is just a "sponger" and accompanies the shoals of shark with the sole object of picking up such crumbs as may fall from their table.

A catfish inhabiting American waters does actually secrete itself within the mouths of giant sharks, and nearer home our own bitterling carp habitually secretes its eggs within the mantle cavity of a big pond mussel where they are hatched and nurtured until the fish have grown big enough to face the world. Many fishes make a practice of sheltering beneath the discs of giant jellyfishes, untouched by the sting-beset tentacles that trail beneath. Here they enjoy abundance of minute food, and complete immunity from hungry foes.

A notorious uninvited guest is the brilliant orange, black and light blue Coral Fish of the East Indies, which lodges within a huge anemone. feeding upon the partially digested food of its invertebrate host. It may be seen swimming about in a little shoal above its strange retreat, but at the slightest hint of danger it at once takes shelter within the gastric cavity of the anemone. There are always a number of these little creatures exhibited in the Zoo Aquarium, where they become very tame and do not require the protection of their former hosts. Unlike most of the aquarium inhabitants which are netted, these coral fish are obtained by native divers who bring up the anemones inside which a specimen is usually to be found.

Another remarkable case of association is that of a small fish which solves its housing problem by living in the body of a sea-cucumber. In this instance the fish leaves the sea-cucumber in the daytime to catch its prey, only returning to its living abode at nightfall.

Crustaceans are notorious both as uninvited guests, and as victims of that unpopular fraternity. The common pea-crab for instance, is always associated with the oyster. The female's shell is so thin as to be a mere membrane and for safety the crab hides in the mantle lobe of the hospitable mollusc. The male, smaller, more active, and better armoured, pays court to his lady in her shelly bower—the oyster permitting. Sometimes this deep-sea Romeo will have to wait for hours on end for the oyster to open and give him access to the bridal chamber.

The hermit crab in his borrowed shell may be seriously hampered by his guests. In addition to carrying two or even three anemones, on the roof of his house, the inside of his shell may be invaded by a large bristle worm that like the human uninvited guest is in great evidence at meal times. Besides this the hermit may have to put up with scores of acorn barnacles, young sponges, and corallines. Some tropical hermit crabs ensconce their tender abdomens in masses of anemones which anchor themselves to the outer cuticle, the crab thus dispensing with a cumbrous borrowed shell. But to see cadging, mendicancy, and shameless dependence on the dole practised to perfection we must go to the insect world. We all know the ancient school-room fable of the ant who refused alms to the thriftless grasshopper. Recent researches show that the ants are exploited and victimized by a hoard of hangers-on. The termites or so-called white ants, raise very ant-like nests, and these harbour a species of bombardier beetle. The beetle can discharge a highly volatile fluid which upon coming into contact with the air explodes with an appreciable report. One such discharge can lay out a large number of ants, dead or stunned, upon their backs. The cunning beetle has learnt, however, that beggars cannot also be bombers, and has suppressed its natural tendency to violence so thoroughly as almost to have lost the faculty. The fleet-footed Thrips, a winged insect common in old houses, is much given to invading ants' nests, relying for safety on its swiftness of foot. It waits until an ant is passing food to a comrade, when it dashes forward and deftly intercepts the morsel. Mites are very common in ants' nests and ride about on the heads of their hosts, convenient situations from which to snatch free meals.

In the nests of some leaf-cutting ants a tiny cockroach is often in evidence. Through living in such close proximity to the ants' ever-busy jaws it eventually parts company with its antennæ. When, therefore, seized with the pangs of hunger and unable to locate the food supply it literally sits up and begs before the nearest ant, who almost invariably provides a dinner.

Many of these professional beggars acquire in the course of countless generations an extraordinary likeness to the insects they habitually victimize. There exists for instance, certain lazy flies that so resemble the humble bees on whom they "sponge" that they enter the hive as they please, being taken by the bees as members of the family.

A certain species of small fly which takes long distance flights without exerting itself to the extent of a single wing beat offers a splendid example of the uninvited guest. When overcome by the desire for travel it just climbs aboard a big night-flying beetle.

CHAPTER X

PUGILISTS

ALL animals, not excluding the human species, can be inspired to fight under such varied stimuli as the tender passions and the fear of death. The lust for wealth is in man another inspiration, and the modern professional pugilist will subject his person to furious assault and battery for often a comparatively paltry prize.

Many different kinds of animals have for centuries been specially bred and trained for the ring, and to this day beasts, birds, fish and even insects are cultivated for the gladiatorial arena.

The ancient Romans staged animal fights—as they staged everything—on a grand scale. Gibbon in his *Decline and Fall of the Roman Empire* gives some amazing statistics of " set pieces " once enjoyed by the rich and poor of ancient Rome. Scores of lions or tigers were pitted against each other at a single performance. On one occasion Nero, anxious to impress the spectators who were already glutted with bloodshed, ordered hundreds of lions, tigers, leopards, bears, hyaenas and wolves to be turned into the arena, and an orgy of carnage ensued which sickened even the blood-drunken audience.

Nearer home and at a much later date animal fights and "baitings" of every kind were extremely popular. In Mr. Pepys' day the bear pit flourished in such quarters as Marylebone and Islington, as many as eight bears being often baited at one time. The bear warden was an honoured personage and held office under the Crown. The carcases of the unfortunate animals were sold for food and barber's grease. The modern bull fight of "cultured" Spain needs no comment. The old English mastiff and bull terrier were both, not so very long ago, in demand as professional pugilists.

Cock-fighting is the only variant of this "sport" still in existence in Great Britain. It not only exists, but has a wide following in the mining districts, many making a good living solely by the training and rearing of fighting cocks. The birds are mostly of the Indian game breed. They are denuded of their combs and wattles and furnished with three-inch steel spurs strapped firmly over the weapons provided by Nature.

"If this don't beat cock-fighting nothing never will, as the Lord Mayor said when the seckertary got up and proposed his misseses health after dinner."

This immortal remark of Mr. Sam Weller's shows how high was the esteem in which cock-fighting was once held throughout Great Britain. Men of every rank, from lord to labourer, kept such cocks as they could afford, and frequently more. Pepys describing a meeting exclaims: "But, Lord, to see the strange variety of people from Parliament men to the poorest prentices, backers, brewers, butchers, dragmen and whatnot." The cockpit was often near to the cathedral or minster and many a church dignitary kept a large stud of cocks with a corresponding staff to tend and train the birds. At the present day cock-fighting commands its maximum popularity in certain South American states. The season lasts from September to June—the birds moulting in the months of July and August. During this period the pugilistic animals roam at large with the hens, care being taken to give each male a run to himself as disputes as to the possession of a bride are liable to have a fatal termination. The training of a fighting cock is no less arduous than that imposed upon a Derby favourite. Having passed through the barber's hands to have its hackles and comb trimmed, the bird is occasionally bathed in rum with the object of discouraging parasites, a procedure which invariably results in the inebriation of the bather. Having recovered from the effects of the bath it is carefully weighed. Should it exceed four pounds it is vigorously exercised. In the early stages of the training the spurs are covered with wadding and an exhaustive course of "seeding" is maintained, until champions worthy of each other are discovered. The best cocks "knock out" at a single blow without holding their opponents by their beaks, "holding" being discouraged as in the human prize ring. The birds are bathed daily in cold water. In the process of drying they are attached to pegs in the sun, and during this period are exercised by the trainer who holds another male bird just within reach. After about fifteen minutes of exercise the pet of the prize ring is massaged and given his one meal of the day, a mess consisting of maize, raw beef, and hard boiled egg. The water ration is reduced by easy stages to a minimum of two mouthfuls a day. On the day of the fight the bird is brought into the ring in a cotton bag, and his owner publicly declares its weight. The pugilists are then hung each at one end of the scale. Very little difference in weight between the birds is allowed, and if one outweighs the other by more than two ounces, another opponent must be found.

Between the rounds the cocks are refreshed by blowing water from the mouth over their heads and necks—a procedure still practised in our own East End boxing rings.

Most birds during the mating season are keen pugilists. The fighting quail of India is a diminutive bird with the ferocity of a tiger, and native farmers of the "fancy" will trek many miles in order to enter their birds at the annual quail tournament. The bird's method of attack is peculiar. Invariably it makes a rush for its adversary's wing, and having established a firm grip applies a screwing pressure that often results in the breakage or dislocation of the wing. The fights between the male ruffs are always a centre of attraction at the Zoo during the month of May. The birds stand facing one another with their shield-like ruffs of feathers encircling the neck erected, and thrust savagely with their long slender beaks. Although appearing very ferocious not much damage results from these duels. But the feathered champion is undoubtedly the talking Mynah of the Indian hill districts. The Mynah, a relation of the crows, locks its feet with those of

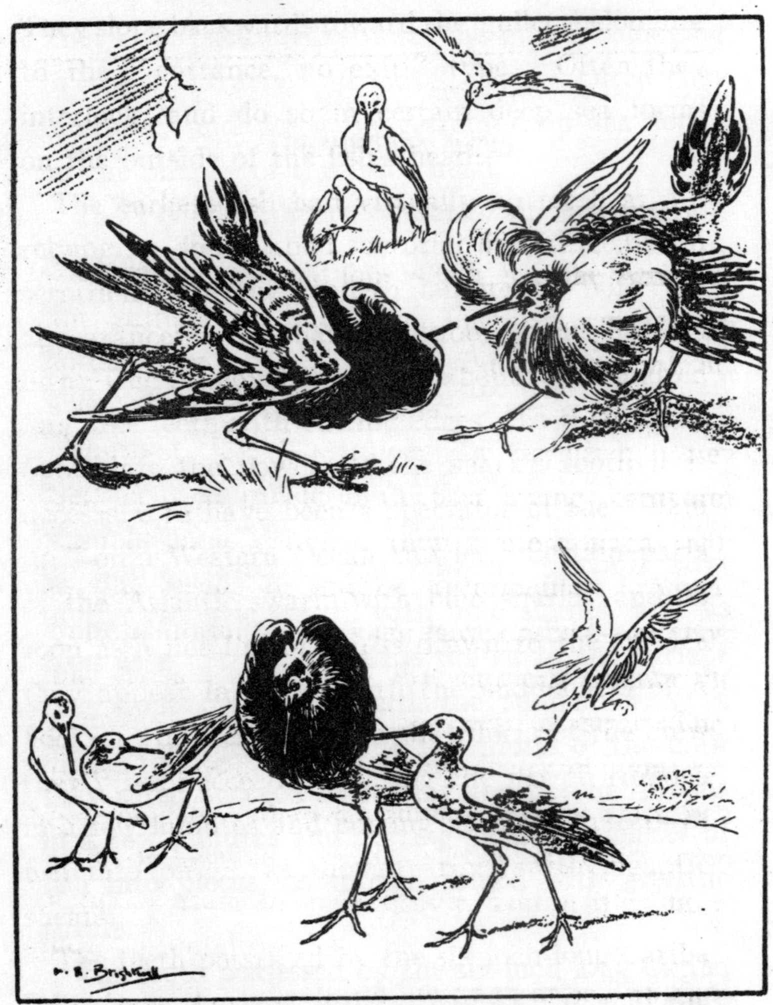

Ruffs during Courtship

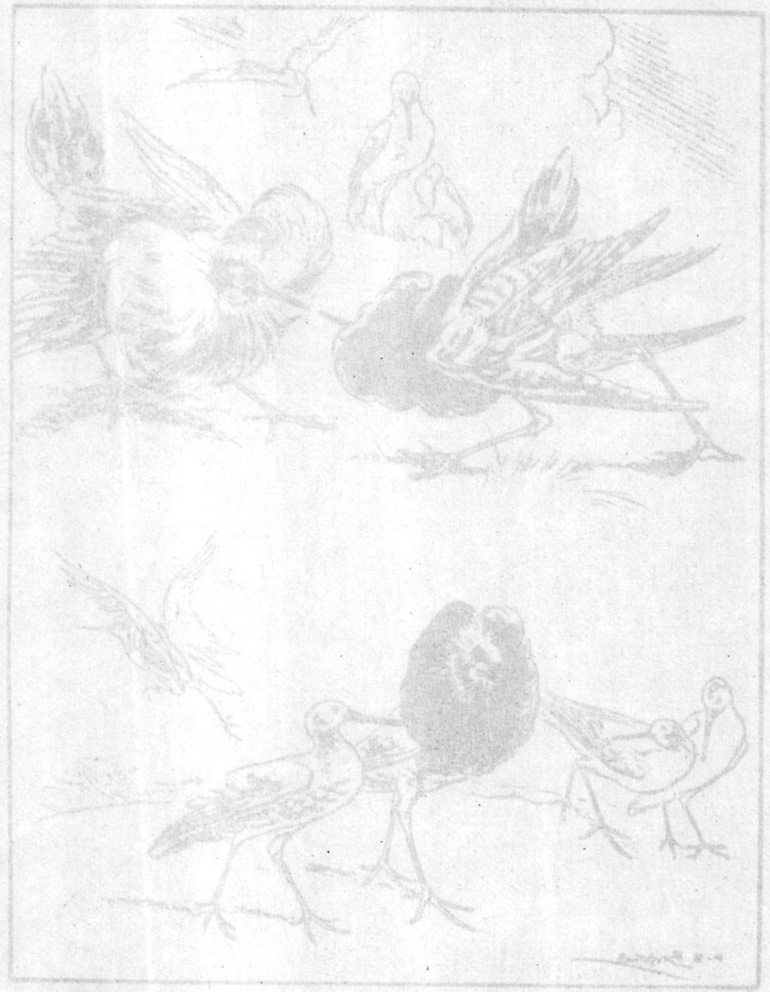

its antagonist and beating the air with its wings employs its beak with lightning rapidity and dagger-like effect.

Elephants are sometimes encouraged to fight one another. In India the two opponents are placed on either side of a mud wall, and make frantic efforts to dislodge the mahouts seated on their necks. Camel fights are promoted annually throughout the Soudan. A hundred or more camels may be drawn up in two ranks facing each other. Down the centre is led a female. At once the flame of conflict is lighted in every male breast. The bull camels are next led two by two into the prize ring where they at once engage. Teeth are sometimes employed but the conflict resolves itself mainly into a grotesque wrestling match, the long and muscular neck being employed as a sort of fifth limb. The fight ends in a "throw."

The pugilistic gifts of the little Fighting Fish are greatly appreciated in the country of its origin, namely, Siam, and the fish outvies all other creatures in the influence which it possesses over man's instinct for gambling. Until a quite recent date the frequenters of these fish fights were wont to stake not only their entire fortunes but their personal liberty and that of their families on the results of these piscatorial contests. Up to the early part of the past century it was a common occurrence for the loser to undergo a long term of slavery to his successful competitor. Fighting Fish tournaments are held all over Siam. The rivals, each measuring under two inches in length, face one another in a large bowl. A round lasts but a few minutes, and so great is the damage entailed that a fish rarely fights more than one round, after which, if he lives, he is relegated to the stud.

An eye-witness account of the savage encounters—regular duels—between rival bees of the same hive has been given by Figuier. "Very hot weather has the effect of irritating the bees, and making them boil over with rage. They are then dangerous to man, whom they attack boldly. But more often it is amongst themselves that they quarrel. One often sees two bees which meet and seize each other by the neck in the air. It happens also that a bee in a state of fury, throws itself on another who is walking quietly and unsuspiciously along the edge of its hive. When two bees are struggling they descend to the ground, for in the air they would not be able to get purchase enough to be sure of striking each other. They then engage in a hand-to-hand fight, as the gladiators used formerly to do in the circus. They are continually making stabs with their stings, but almost always the point slips over the scales with which they are covered. The combat may be prolonged during an hour before one of them has found the weak point in the other's natural cuirass, and has buried its terrible weapon in the flesh. The victor often leaves its sting in the wound which it has made and then dies in its moment of triumph through the loss of this organ. Sometimes the two combatants, in spite of long and savage assaults, cannot succeed in injuring either's solid armour. In such a case they leave each other, tired of war, and fly away, despairing of obtaining a victory."

The natives of certain parts of China, hard put to it for some means of indulging their sporting tastes, find a good and cheap substitute in the Praying Mantis, and the insects are made to fight one another in public. The quarrelsome creatures need no encouragement, and will attack their own kind on the slightest provocation, the conqueror invariably devouring his antagonist.

Fighting proclivities have sometimes led to an extraordinary development of some particular feature—claws, horns, or tusks. In the age of Reptiles a huge dinosaur—Triceratops—developed an excess of armature which eventually led to its extinction. It became so unwieldy that it was unable to cope with smaller but more active and intelligent competitors, and the animal has gone down to posterity as an awful example of over-specialization.

CHAPTER XI

ARCHITECTS

HUMAN architecture must have had its birth when man first decided that the cave might be improved upon as a desirable residence. But the wild-animal world anticipated architecture, as it anticipated flight and wireless many millions of years before the first human stonemason or bricklayer came into being. Architecture is to-day applied solely to the art of planning and designing a building, but in its original form the word embraced not only the planning but also the major portion of the constructing. In the animal world every architect is likewise a builder, for all creatures desiring homes of their own creation must not only plan but construct.

The fact that the animals most nearly akin to man show the least aptitude for the architectural profession is one of the many anomalies of Nature. Very few mammals, for instance, hanker after an "ideal home," being usually content with a ready-made hollow in the ground, a burrow, an overhanging rock-shelf, a cave, or a simple clearing in thick grass or undergrowth. One of man's nearest relatives—the orang-utan—is, however, an exception, for it constructs a platform of twigs and another a few feet above it which serves as a roof. The most popular form of mammalian architecture is the burrow. The badger will dig down through sixteen feet of solid chalk, whilst the male water-rat excavates underground fortresses showing much cunning and design.

The beaver is in a class by itself, its strongly-built lodges—huge structures composed of wood and mud—being superior in both design and construction to many a native hut. The beaver will work night and day for months on end, regarding eight hours a day as a ridiculously short spell. In the summer of 1916 observation was kept on a party of ten Canadian beavers that had embarked upon the construction of a lodge. When fairly started on their work two of the builders were swept away by autumnal floods. Storms and floods subsequently killed two more and carried three of the survivors some miles from the half-erected home. Yet the lodge was established and made proof against the severest weather before the winter had fairly closed in.

The architectural attempts of the members of

the feathered world are still more bewildering. A few birds are content with a mere depression in the ground, but the majority give up months of labour to the making of the home, and in its erection employ an enormous variety of materials. Many of the finches build nests by binding leaves together with fibre, or construct flask-shaped nests suspended beneath umbrellas of sticks and straw—secure alike from snake and tempest. Others combine to form what are literally aerial flats—immense ganglions of fibre-built nests, all linked together, yet each nest pleasantly isolated from its neighbour. The most æsthetic builders are the Australian bower-birds, each different species having its own particular conception of what "art in the home" should be like. In the construction of the bowers one kind may use nothing but wool and cotton; another may prefer shells and feathers; whilst yet a third may specialize in brightly-coloured flowers, which, when they begin to wither are immediately renewed.

Birds are truly adaptable creatures. An English blackbird has been known to build its home entirely out of old watch springs stolen from an adjacent store, whilst during the War it was not uncommon to find sparrows' nests built in barbed wire entanglements, and consisting chiefly of "precious" Army forms. Equal ingenuity is shown by birds in the handling of clay and mortar.

The widely distributed baker-birds, for instance, build oval-shaped structures of clay, planted in the most blatant manner in a perfectly exposed position, where they are taken to be lumps of stone by the hungry night-prowling beasts. These clay nests take many months to construct, and become so hard that a hammer must be employed to extract the eggs.

The cock hornbill annually incarcerates his lady in a hollow tree and bricks up the opening with clay, leaving a space sufficient for the passing in of the food.

Reptiles which are so closely related to birds, are disappointing as architects, and their entire inability to construct homes other than burrows must for ever remain a mystery. Even the burrow is usually annexed, ready-made, the result of much labour on the part of some industrious mammal or bird.

Many amphibians—frogs, toads, etc.—protect their young by building elaborate nests and nurseries. Thus a large Brazilian tree-frog erects a basin-shaped nursery in the shallow waters of the borders of the ponds it frequents during the breeding season. The mud is scooped out by the female to a depth of three or four inches, and with the material thus removed she builds a circular wall. The frog during this operation employs its flat-webbed feet for smoothing the inside of the parapet in exactly the same manner that a mason uses his trowel.

The members of the fish tribe number many proficient architects, amongst which the stickle-back or " tiddler " takes pride of place. The nests are usually very bird-like in pattern, and are built upon the sea or river beds. They are com-posed of weeds bitten off into suitable lengths, and poked together with the snout, which is used as a pile-driver. Sometimes a salivary secretion is used to bind the mass together.

Almost every known building material—other than metal and asbestos—is employed by insects. The teeming termites of Africa and Australia raise enormous nests strong enough to bear tremendous weights. Wood pulp was turned into paper by wasps millions of years before man was evolved. Wax is to the bee what clay is in the hands of a skilled potter, whilst the strength and weather-resisting qualities of silk are clearly demonstrated in many widely separated depart-ments of the insect world, where the commodity is used in lieu of carpets, roofing, and wallpapers.

The larvæ of the caddis fly construct remarkable tubular houses from shells, gravel, and sticks. They are very entertaining to watch when placed in a small aquarium, especially when provided with coloured beads, which they will use for the construction of their homes with the most dazzling effects.

The architectural attainments of bees are very marvellous, their homes as a rule being destined not only to be an abode but also a food store. The Carpenter Bee hollows out deep galleries in wood, and builds in them regular shaped cells. After the main structure has been formed and the egg laid in a mass of pollen mixed with honey, the cell is closed by forming a ceiling of sand agglutinated with saliva. On this ceiling a new cell is established, and so the work goes on between intervals of egg-laying.

The Mason Bee builds massive irregular-shaped nests against the sides of walls and houses. A suitable sunny spot having been chosen, the bee flies off in search of building material, and collects sand and small pebbles which she mixes with a little earth and her saliva. The mortar thus formed becomes very hard and is fixed on the chosen site, but not until sufficient material has been gathered does she start on the complicated structures of the regular-shaped cells. Finally a roof of coarse sand is fixed over this very substantial abode.

The Leaf-Cutting Bees build tubular homes lined with leaves, the nest consisting of about five cells. The pieces of leaf are cut off with the creatures' mandibles, and the notches thus formed are as clearly cut as if they had been punched by a machine.

The Upholsterer Bees are even more romantic, lining their burrows with the petals of flowers. The abodes contain but a single cell which when the egg has been laid is filled up with earth to prevent detection.

The tough paper-like homes of wasps, formed of fibre mixed with saliva, are usually built on the ground. A gallery a foot or more long leads to the nest which is composed of fifteen or sixteen horizontal galleries arranged in storeys and supported by pillars. The nest has been aptly described as a small subterranean town surrounded by a wall, in which the streets and dwelling-places are perfectly regularly distributed. In the building of "wasp town" wood fibre forms the principal raw material. The fibre is made into balls which are carried between the legs of the insects to the nest, where after being stuck together they are flattened out and drawn into thin layers, in the manner employed by a bricklayer when spreading mortar with a trowel.

The Card-Making Wasp of Cayenne is so called from the fact that its abode represents a box composed of a white cardboard-like substance.

The nests of ants are elaborate structures. Figuier has given a detailed description of their homes: "Each species has an order of architecture peculiar to it. The Red Ant, one of the commonest in our woods, constructs a little rounded hillock with all kinds of objects—fragments of wood, bits of straw, dry leaves, the remains of insects, etc. This hillock, whose base is protected by material of greater solidity, is nothing more than the exterior envelope of the nest which is carried underground to a very great depth. Avenues, cleverly contrived, lead from the summit to the interior. The openings vary in width, and as night approaches are carefully barricaded. They are opened every morning except on rainy days when the doors remain shut and the inhabitants confined within.

"The ant-hill, or formicarium, is at first simply a hole hollowed out in the soil, the entrance to which is masked by the building materials. But the miners do not cease to hollow out galleries and chambers arranged by storeys. The earth and rubbish are carried out, and serve to construct the upper edifice, which rises at the same time that the excavation grows deeper. It is a labyrinth bored in all directions. It contains corridors, landings, chambers, and spacious rooms which communicate with each other by passages which are often vertical. All the corridors lead to a large central space, loftier than the others, and supported by pillars; it is here that the greater number of the ants congregate. These ant-hills often rise to a height of fifteen inches above the ground, and descend to an equal depth.

"The large group of Mason Ants all employ a mortar in the construction of their hills. The masons work when they can profit by the rain or by the evening dew to make their mortar. They only go out after sunset, or when fine rain has wetted their roof. Then they set to work. They roll up pellets of earth, bring them back in their mandibles, and stick them on to those places where the building was left unfinished. From all sides the workers may be seen arriving, laden with materials. All these are bustling, hurrying, busy, but always in the greatest order, and with a perfect understanding among themselves. Every part of the building is going on at the same time.

The apartments spring up one above another, and the edifice visibly rises. The rain, the sun, and the wind consolidate and harden the building so cunningly contrived by these industrious workers. With no other tool than their mandibles, the excavators work their way through the hardest wood. They bore holes right through it, riddling it completely with numerous storeys of horizontal galleries. Independent of the principal entrances there exist in some nests, masked doors guarded by sentinels. Many species also hollow out covered galleries, which they only unmask in extreme danger, either to open an outlet for the besieged, or to turn the enemy who has already invaded the place. Ant-hills are in fact perfect fortresses, defended by a thousand ingenious devices, and guarded by sentinels always on the *qui vive*."

The much dreaded ant-like creatures known as Termites build enormous edifices. The colonies living in these structures consist of workers measuring about one-fifth of an inch in length, the slightly larger soldiers, distinguished by their enormous heads armed with large pincers, the normal males, and the six-inch long females whose abdomens when about to lay become two thousand times as large as the rest of their bodies. The lady termite's fecundity is astounding, laying at the rate of eighty thousand eggs a day for several months in the year. A pregnant female, although only an inch or so longer than a worker, weighs as much as thirty thousand workers.

The nests, composed chiefly of wood stuck together with a gum, may measure twenty feet in height and are almost as disproportionate to the size of the inhabitants as is the Woolworth Building in New York. Certain termites raise columns which support a large flat abode, giving the structures the appearance of a gigantic mushroom. The columns are constructed of clay which worked up by the insects acquire very great hardness. So solid are the houses of the Central African termites that not only can men mount on them without doing any damage, but buffaloes have been known to make use of them as watch towers from which to look out for approaching enemies.

The edifices are hollow but the sides are hard as rock. Under the central dome is a large space occupying nearly one third of the total height. On the ground floor is the royal cell with a rounded ceiling and pierced with numbers of small round windows. All round are the workers' offices — rooms with vaulted ceilings communicating with each other by passages. On the sides are the stores in which the various juices are kept. Just above the queen's chamber are the egg-rooms—small cells with walls composed of sawdust mixed with gum. Finally between the royal cell and the central dome is the nursery, the best site of all and specially chosen for its uniformity of temperature.

The elaborate subterranean homes of certain crickets are not to be despised, especially those of the Mole Cricket which makes use of its spade-shaped hands for excavating numerous horizontal galleries. Like those of the mammal from which it derives its name, the abode is always recognizable by the mounds of rubbish which are heaped up at the sides of the front door.

Spiders build delicate silky homes to which they often become much attached. In the black and yellow Signature Spiders of the South of France the middle of the web is crossed by a zig-zag band of white silk—the so-called "Signature"—which, as the web is obliquely hung, conceals the spider beneath it. These and other spiders repair their webs by tearing out old and dirty pieces and replacing them by new ones. One species raises a cylindrical tower and builds a dome-like roof over it made of a web overlaid with leaves. The whole is fastened down except

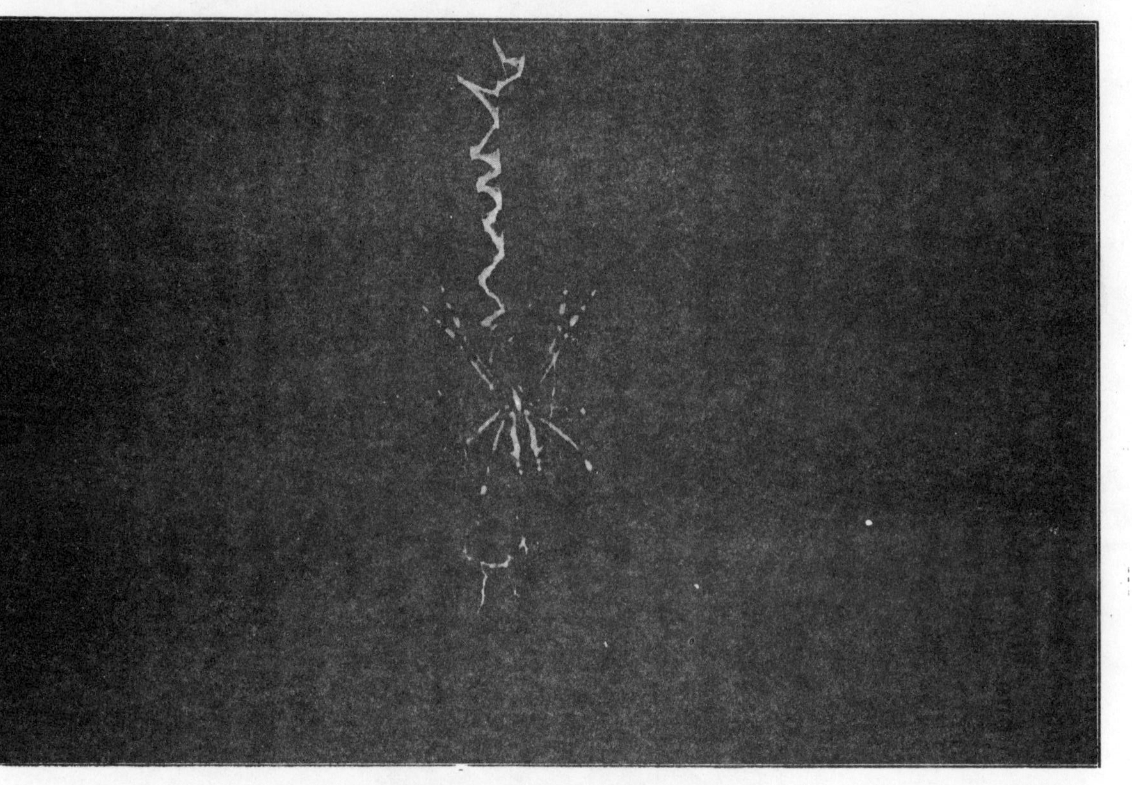

THE SIGNATURE SPIDER.

[p. 132.

for a small entrance and exit which remains hermetically sealed during the winter months and on such occasions as their wasp enemies are engaged in provisioning raids.

The crafty West African Trap-Door Spider builds a rainproof abode, a structure serving the dual purpose of excluding enemies and keeping the rain out. The home consists of a tubular excavation lined with silk with the two ends closed by a hinged door composed of leaves and earth. One of the doors is constantly used but the other serves only in case of emergency. On an enemy attempting to enter by the front door, the spider attempts to keep it closed by holding on with its claws. In the event of failure, however, an escape is effected by the "emergency exit." When only a few weeks old the precocious babies leave the parental roof and sally out into the world to build similar homes of their own.

The aquatic Raft Spider, which may be observed on the surface of most ponds in this country, gathers together dry leaves, twigs and rubbish and binds them together with silk to form a raft on which it may be blown about the water. The still more aquatic Diving-Bell Spider works under water where it constructs a soft silky cup-shaped sac, having an opening on the under surface.

Into this opening air bubbles are introduced, each bubble being brought separately from the surface and placed within the miniature diving bell, until completely inflated. Within this strange dwelling the spider spends the best years of its life, and rears a family in a second and quite separate chamber—a nursery within the main structure.

Many molluscs and marine worms employ cement to form long tubular dwellings, continually placing layer upon layer of cement upon the rim of the tube until the structure reaches several feet in length.

Finally, amongst certain minute organisms crowding every spoonful of water—fresh, brackish, or salt—we may note the birth of brickmaking. These miscroscopic creatures build their castles brick by brick in circular tiers, thus forming a house that exactly keeps pace with its owner's steadily increasing requirements, and the mere human, harassed by house-agents, architects, builders, and all they involve, may be excused for envying their remarkable accomplishments.

CHAPTER XII

ANGLERS

THE " gentle art " like most other human activities is not necessarily a human monopoly. It was in fact practised by the lower animals millions of years before the first man attempted to discover a speedier and more efficacious way of obtaining fish than by merely waiting for the receding tide to leave a few chance individuals stranded.

Nets were used by the earliest spiders, the rod was employed by certain cannibal fishes, whilst the spear came into vogue with the first birds. " Tickling " was developed into a fine art by a host of mammals.

Beginning at the top of the scale, monkeys are known to catch fish by the latter method, and certain ancient Egyptian paintings lend colour to the theory that baboons were at one time trained as professional fishermen.

The feline dislike of getting wet is well-known, but the cat's antipathy to water is counter-balanced by its passion for a meal of fish, to gratify which the animal is prepared to brave almost anything, even water. All known species of wild cats that live within reasonable distance of fish-stocked waters are good disciples of Izaak Walton. The Indian Fishing Cat has earned its popular name by its dexterity in sweeping unsuspecting fish ashore, whilst the large and intelligent Jaguar has improved on this method and has been known to lure the fish to their doom by gently waving its tail to and fro in the water. The Canadian lynx not being blessed with a tail of respectable proportions relies solely upon a sudden grab, or even a header to obtain its most coveted dish. Bengal tigers frequenting the banks of the Lower Ganges are sometimes compelled in flood-time to take to the trees and there they rely for sustenance upon a fish menu that involves many a ducking. By far the most interesting examples of fishing cats, however, are found amongst the smug house-pets of everyday life, and scores of instances might be quoted of cats accompanying fishermen —both salt and fresh-water—and sharing the catch which they help to augment. A notable example is that of a big black " Tom " that many years ago accompanied a " longshore " fisherman at Broadstairs. This cat would leap into the sea and capture such swiftly swimming fish as bass and mackerel, and climb aboard with his catch—often nearly as large as himself, lashing wildly between his jaws.

Diving cats are often found attached to mills employing water-power. The cats originally introduced to catch mice, presently wander further afield and acquire a taste for water rats. This pursuit naturally leads to a close acquaintance with fish, and very soon the keen feline wits are at work upon the problem of transferring the fish from the stream bed to their interiors. One such cat would deliberately follow trout along the bank until the quarry came to rest. Then a sudden plunge and the fish was caught.

Cats carried by merchant ships cruising in Southern waters frequently enjoy a meal of flying-fish. The fish as they fly aboard at night are pounced upon by the cat who has been sitting close to the rail on the windward side eagerly awaiting such chance comers. That the fish are attracted by the gleaming eyes of the ship's cat is a sailor's theory, which is almost as difficult to believe in as to verify.

The dog is not nearly as efficient a fisherman as the cat. Its wild ancestors were inhabitants of comparatively dry districts and so mav have failed to acquire the feline's piscatorial skill through lack of opportunity. On certain coasts of the South Seas, however, dogs are trained to catch fish, being employed by the natives to round up the shoals and drive them towards the shore, whilst less than a hundred years ago they were similarly used in Devonshire to round up salmon into nets placed in tidal rivers. Some curious instances of dog fishermen come from our own country. At the beginning of the last century the Earl of Home had a dog that would kill twenty large salmon in a morning, and always on an adjacent estate. This led to a long and costly lawsuit, judgment eventually being given for the dog. There is also a record of a dog living on the coast of Newfoundland that would pile up as many as seventy large fish in the course of a day, each taken alive from deep water. Whilst the cat invariably fishes with an end in view, the dog, having no predilection for a fish dinner, does so in a more light-hearted spirit, and purely *pour le sport*.

Whenever possible man has turned an animal's natural instincts to his own account, and the efforts made in Japan to divert the cormorant's penchant for catching fish into commercial channels has met with a certain measure of success. The cormorants are taken out in batches, each having a ring round its neck to prevent the fish travelling too far down. The birds dive for the fish and being unable to swallow their catch, bring it on board confident of a reward. They not only act as collectors but also as sheep dogs, rounding up the shoals into a small compass. The cormorants are caught young and carefully trained, and a reliable bird is worth a small fortune to its owner.

Fishing birds generally adopt methods that have been approved by man, the method employed being dictated by the creature's form and structure. Thus birds that rely upon spearing their fish show a great development of beak which ends in a sharp point whilst the neck behind it is long and flexible, serving the purpose of a rope attached to a fish-spear or harpoon. The familiar heron is a good example. With a Job-like patience it will remain perfectly still and silent for hours on end, waiting for a chance to strike some unwary victim deceived into mistaking the bird's breast for the sky above and its legs for the reeds of the river bank. Occasionally herons will spear bigger fish than they can comfortably land, and instances are known of their being choked by large trout and strangled by giant eels transfixed beyond all loosening on the needle-pointed beak.

The Darters, nearly related to the professional fishing cormorants, carry the harpoon method still further. The neck is constructed on a "spring trigger" principle, so that the bird literally shoots its quarry—just as the Andaman Islander still shoots his fish with bow and arrow. Like the arrow-head the darter's bill is jagged, being set with many fine serrations, and the beak has been known to have been driven over half an inch into a deal board. Whereas the cormorant swallows its catch under water, the darter invariably brings it to the surface before devouring it.

In the pelican we have a wonderful example of the manner Nature can combine not only the harpoon and rope, but also the landing net, up to 40 lbs. of fish being occasionally held in the bird's enormous membranous throat-pouch before being transferred to its interior.

The Gannet is another well-known feathered fisherman of these islands and terrifying statistics of its fish destroying powers have been compiled. It is doubtful, however, if any feathered animal can be considered a serious competitor with man's all-embracing trawl and trammel nets, and, though a few fishing birds have a price upon their heads, the majority are respected and valued by the fishermen as reliable guides to approaching shoals.

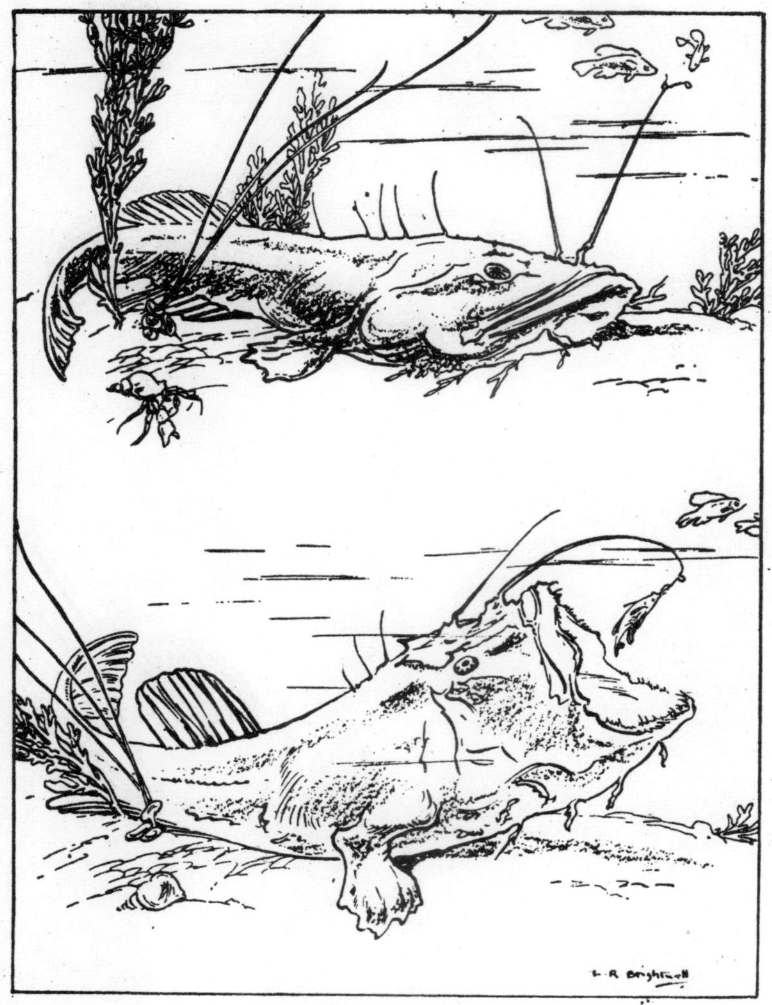

ANGLER FISH

The majority of reptilian fishermen display little imagination. An exception is the Matamata Turtle of the Amazon River, whose rough and irregularly shaped shell often covered with vegetable growth exactly resembles some submerged boulder, an appearance of use to the creature when fishing for its dinner. The most remarkable feature of the Matamata, however, is its chin, this portion of its anatomy being provided with a number of worm-like appendages. This living bait serves the purpose of attracting the unsuspecting fish which fall victims to the " whisker trap " before they have had time to realize their mistake.

Fish, with a few exceptions, live upon fish. Some like the cariba and the sharks tear fragments from the living animals, but the majority swallow their victims entire, and the fish feeding on the stream or sea floor may be regarded as living trawls. The British Angler Fish, however, scorns the trawl and is an enthusiast of rod and line. The " Angler " is a huge lumpish creature growing to five feet in length and often weighing 50 lbs., without its dinner, which on occasions may amount to more than its own weight. The first dorsal fin ray, inserted on the snout, is very long and rod-like, is movable in every direction and terminates in a fleshy flap which is used as a bait, attracting other fishes. When waving in the water this flap of skin looks remarkably like some small fish, so much so indeed that sooner or later it is seized by a passing bass or codling. At once the "rod" bends towards the huge cavernous tooth-rimmed mouth. Once past those teeth there is no returning. His vast gullet acts in a similar manner to the pelican's pouch, as a landing net, and the catch is passed at leisure direct from the landing net to the dinner table in the "Angler's" interior. Angler fish inhabit nearly all seas, and show a wonderful capacity for adapting themselves to any given environment. Usually the breast fins are developed into arm-like appendages, with which the fish stealthily shuffles over the sea-floor, and invariably the creature is arrayed in numerous seaweed-like skinny appurtenances, that harmonize perfectly with its surroundings. Anglers inhabiting the abyssal depth of the oceans have the "lure" illuminated by a phosphorescent bulb, and some of these deep sea anglers devour fish several times their own size, their skins stretching in an accommodating fashion beyond the glutton's wildest dreams.

In a recently discovered angler fish the male has become degenerate and parasitic upon the female, his whole life being spent attached to her by means of a special outgrowth of the head. The disparity in size between the two sexes is very remarkable, the bulky bride weighing twenty pounds or more whilst the consort is so small as to be barely visible to the naked eye. Most curious, however, is the fact that he derives all his nourishment from his wife to whom he is grafted and whose blood supply he shares.

Another method, and a very effectual one indeed, deserves mention—the use of electricity. The Electric Eel of the Amazon River and the Electric Ray or Torpedo of our shores both catch their food by "shocking" it into insensibility. The manner in which the small Electric Catfish of the rivers of Tropical East Africa makes use of its electric powers is slightly different. Swimming slowly alongside a much larger fish it creates a contact by deliberately touching its quarry. The shock is not powerful enough to kill, but sufficient to force the victim to bring up any half-digested food stored inside him, which the perpetrator of this disgusting outrage remains behind to enjoy at his leisure.

The electric organs of the eel and the ray are derived from modifications of the muscular tissue, but those of the catfish are developed from the glandular system. Although the currents created exercise all the properties of electricity, decomposing certain chemical compounds and emitting sparks, in spite of much careful investigation no satisfactory explanation has yet been given of the phenomenon.

Many insects and spiders are expert fishermen. Mr. Wallace Adams of the Steinhardt Aquarium, at San Francisco has given an account of a spider catching fish: "We had a number of Pigmy Sunfish in one of the aquaria in our swamp room. The specimens kept disappearing in a most unaccountable manner until one morning I found the remains of two in a fold of an overhanging leaf in which a spider had made a nest." The giant "edible" water bug of Mexico deliberately hounds down fish full of vigour, whilst some of the wolf spiders actually construct silken rafts on which they punt about the sluggish waters and catch small fish basking near the surface.

Amongst the mollusca only the cuttlefish can be regarded as fishermen, and they employ a very ingenious method to entrap their catches. Two long sucker-tipped arms which when at rest are tucked away into pockets in the head, are "run out" when a fish is sighted and the saucer-shaped suckers covering the club-shaped tip at once attach themselves with a deadly hold. This use of the "sucker" has been imitated by man, for in certain parts of the South Seas sucking fishes (Remora) attached to lines are put over the side of vessels, and the fishes given all the freedom they desire till they affix themselves to a shark or turtle, when the line is hauled in and the Remora again liberated for another catch.

The angling methods of that cucumber-shaped relative of the starfish—the Cotton Spinner—are noteworthy, the creature ejecting vast quantities of sticky threads which swell on exposure in the water and form an entanglement from which a fish or crab seldom succeeds in escaping.

One worm at least is an habitual fisherman. This is the "living fishing line" the Nemertes—a common British sea-worm measuring anything from a few inches to 90 feet in length. The "line" when reeled in, i.e., quiescent, resembles a solid lump of calf's liver. Should, however, a fish come within touch of its suctorial mouth, a marvellous transformation takes place, the lump of "liver" revealing itself as a long unbreakable line that "plays" the fish until the energies of the latter are exhausted. The tail of Brer Fox who went fishing by hanging his tail over the edge of a pond is sufficiently extravagant, but as we have seen it is easily outclassed by what actually occurs in Nature—yet another tribute to the truth of the platitude: "Fact is stranger than fiction."

CHAPTER XIII

CAMOUFLAGE

THE word camouflage literally translated implies a puff of smoke blown into the face, therefore an affront; but the meaning of the term has in recent years been stretched to embrace " blinds " and concealments of all kinds. During the Great War the various armies gave detailed attention to this question of camouflage, and resorted to nature for their sources of information. Guns were painted to resemble mossy banks and bushes, tents and huts were coaxed to melt into the landscape, and ships were made to emulate various surface-haunting creatures that, owing to their wavy patterns, were inconspicuous even to the trained observer. This idea of camouflage was practised by the most primitive races, who screened themselves with bushes when advancing to meet the enemy, just as the Kaffirs to this day when stalking ostriches disguise themselves in the skins of the birds.

But to see camouflage in perfection we must

visit the animal world, for those creatures that do not practise the art of concealment are in a very small minority. Brilliant colours are often the surest means of camouflage, although occasionally we find them so assorted that they are conspicuous amid any surroundings. They may then be regarded as warnings. The wasp's gay stripes and the porcupine's striking livery of black and white both spell " beware," whilst the skunk's jazzy costume calls out " go away —or be gassed." Many strikingly marked caterpillars taste so unpleasant that no bird meddles with them twice.

Quite a number of harmless creatures have found that it pays to adopt the warning colours of certain dangerous animals, and thus perfectly innocuous flies are attired to look like wasps, and defenceless rodents are dressed to resemble pugnacious shrews. These delicate cases of flattery are, however, not very common, and most animals seek protection in assimilating the colour of their environment. The algae covering the hide of ancient crocodiles and the lichens draping the long-haired sloths are disguises which lend their wearers adequate protection. Sometimes the camouflage takes the form of a direct imitation of the surroundings, and, especially amongst in-

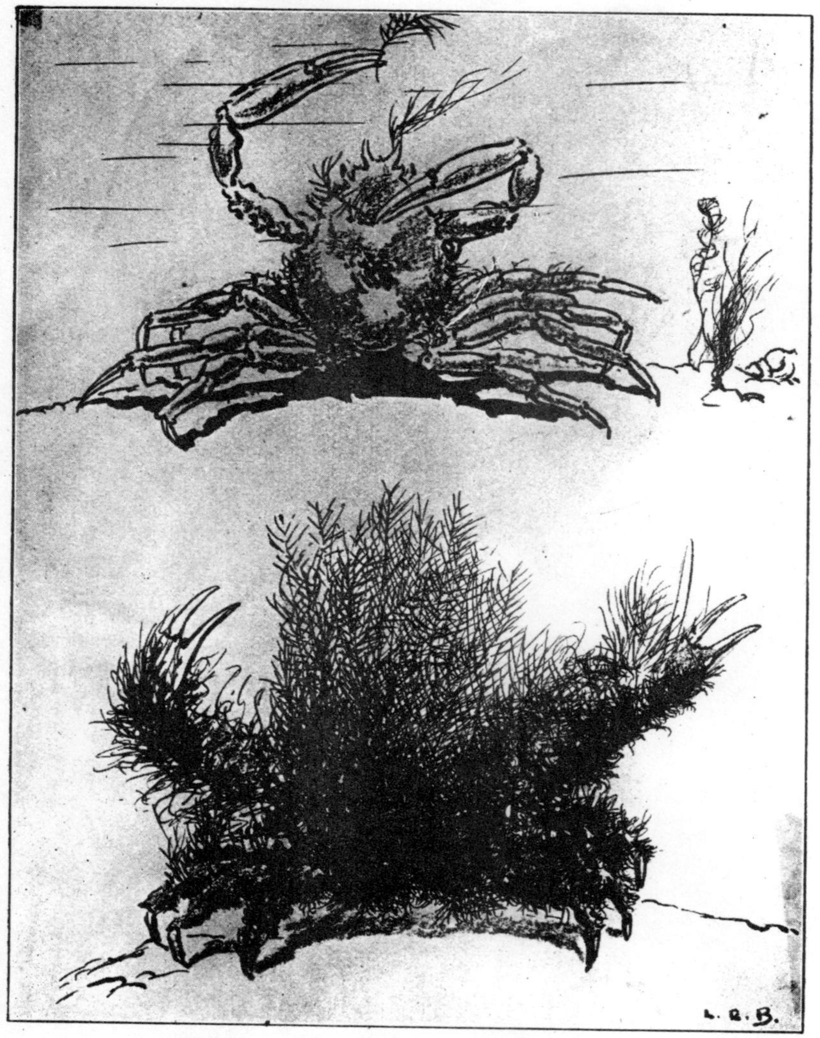

SPIDER CRAB (DRESSED AND UNDRESSED).

[p. 150.

vertebrates, there are many instances of creatures desirous of shunning the limelight deliberately "dressing up" for the purpose. The members of the family of spider crabs attire their rugged shells with weeds, corallines, shells, and heaps of débris. Often the weeds take root amongst the dense growth of hooked hairs covering the carapace and limbs. Should the crab not change its shell for some time, the weeds flourish until the crustacean resembles a miniature forest. A few spider crabs have shells that are not covered with a stiff scrub of hooked bristles, and are ill-adapted for giving anchorage to weeds and corallines. Instead, their shells show a porous, pipe-clayed surface, which makes an ideal site for sponges to grow upon. The hermit crab's habit of tucking its defenceless tail into empty shells is purely a matter of safety first, rather than an ingenious form of camouflage. One hermit, however, instead of hiding its nether portion in a shell, covers this part of its anatomy with a mass of sea anemones, thus not only enjoying their protection, but often sharing in their "catch." The disguise in certain members of the insect world is used with the object of concealment and of attracting prey. A remarkable example of what has been called "Alluring Coloration" is that of a bright pink wingless Mantis inhabiting the forests of India. Its large abdomen is shaped like the labellum of an orchid whilst the thighs and posterior legs are dilated to resemble the petals of a blossom. When motionless amidst green foliage with the thorax and abdomen at right angles to one another and with the fore legs hidden and the back legs stretched out, it forms a perfect replica of a flower. As a result of this mimicry unsuspecting insects are attracted to the mantis, settle upon it in the belief that it really is an orchid and are promptly captured and devoured. Another Indian mantis, Songlees, resembles a flower and thereby secures a very handsome living by deceiving insects. The under surface of this creature is coloured either white, violet or mauve, and acquires a reddish tinge towards the margins so as to resemble a flower with a white or a purple corolla. In the centre is a blackish brown blotch which is exactly like the opening of a tube in the middle of a flower. So perfect is the floral resemblance in this case that the practised eyes of botanists have been deceived. The resemblance of certain insects to the excreta of birds is another instance of aggressive resemblance, certain flies being known to be attracted by the droppings. A small British crab—the

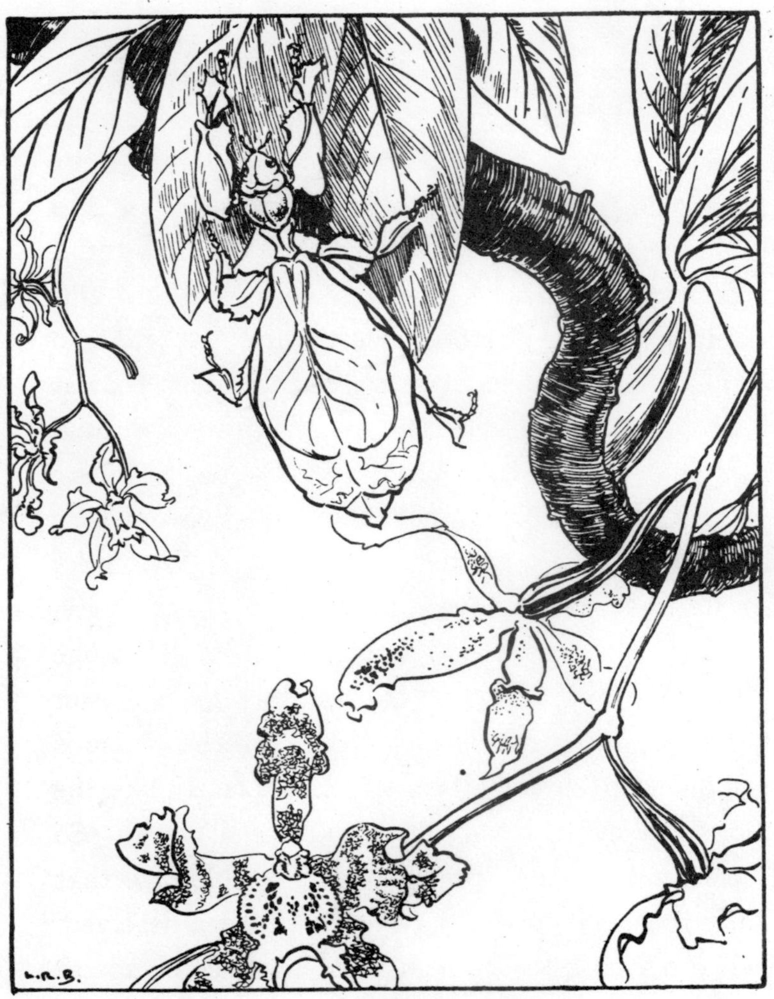

Leaf Insect

sponge crab, common on West Country oyster beds—habitually holds a large sponge over its back with one claw, the sponge often being five or six times as large as the crab. A certain bug in the pupa stage—before the wings are developed, resembles a specially ugly spider. It is enveloped with a thick greyish matter which is nothing but the dust mixed with wool, cloth, etc., which congregates in badly-swept rooms. Under this borrowed costume the insect is just twice its real size. By means of this masquerade it is able to approach the flies upon which it preys. When stripped the little creature presents the appearance of a totally different animal, and is tolerably good looking.

The insect world offers many other cases of camouflage. The best examples are those curious relations of the cockroach, the leaf insects, which so exactly resemble the leaves of the plants they live on that they are almost impossible to detect when stationary. The wings of the creatures cover almost their entire bodies, and resemble leaves not only in shape, but in the fact that their veins are so disposed as to imitate exactly the prominent ribs present on the leaves of plants. The colour of these insects is bright green, but when dying most specimens pass through the different dull hues of a decaying leaf. The eggs of the leaf insect so strongly resemble the seeds of certain plants than even experienced botanists are deceived by the similarity. A few butterflies likewise resemble leaves, mimicking their form and colouring. A good example is that of a large species inhabiting Northern India whose upper sides are the dull brown of a dead leaf with darker veins. As a result an amazing transforming takes place when the creature settles on a bush, for within a fraction of a second a brilliantly adorned butterfly is changed as if by magic into a withered leaf.

The stick insects and stick caterpillars are other well-known classical examples. Dr. Wallace has described the stick insects in the Moluccas "hanging on shrubs that line the forest paths, they resemble sticks so exactly in colour, in small rugosities of the bark, in the knots and small branches imitated by the joints of legs which are either pressed close to the body or stuck out at random, that it is absolutely impossible by the eye alone to distinguish the real dead twigs which fall down from the trees overhead from the living insects. Often," he states, "I have looked at them in doubt and have been obliged to use the sense of touch to determine the point."

Of the many caterpillars that likewise resemble sticks those known as the Geometers are most remarkable. They may be observed embracing the stem of a twig or leaf with their hinder legs whilst the rest of their body is vertically elevated. In such an attitude they will remain stiff and motionless for hours on end. Less famous are certain sociable caterpillars of Tropical Africa, which cluster round a twig so as to resemble a notoriously poisonous berry eschewed by bird and beast alike. Of the several hundred species of moths found in Great Britain quite two-thirds harmonize perfectly with the subdued marbling of the moss and fungus mottled woodland trees. Everywhere this tendency to blend with the background is apparent. The hare and grouse are one with the moorland heath and bracken; the gull's eggs are indistinguishable from the pebbles constituting the nest, whilst the creatures emanating from desert lands are with very few exceptions clad in khaki suits. Not that a dress of similar tint to the immediate surroundings is a guaranteed cloak of invisibility. Strong light may cast heavy shadows on the creature's underside and cause it to stand out in strong relief. To counteract this most animals are coloured darker above and lighter beneath, thus nullifying the "relief" that would otherwise give them away.

In countries where vivid sunlight is the rule, Nature employs all kinds of devices to break up the outer surface of an animal in order to make it blend with the check pattern of sunlit grass and foliage. The tiger's stripes and the giraffe's spots are but two of many hundreds of instances that might be quoted.

A most effective form of camouflage is seen in those creatures that can change their colours or markings at will. For some reason the chameleon has attained a world-wide reputation as Nature's champion "quick change" artist. Actually he is often rather slow to alter his colouring to meet a change in his surroundings. There is an old story of a chameleon that burst when placed upon a Highland plaid. Certainly many other creatures would be undaunted by such a test and have no difficulty in accomplishing the feat. The American anolis and the Indian changeable lizard are much more adept at a sudden transformation than any chameleon. Exhaustive experiments with fishes have shown that the plaice and turbot can at short notice accommodate themselves to almost any pattern however intricate. The world's quick-change championship is probably held by the octopus, which can, whilst striding spider-like across the sea-bed, alter its tints to suit each succeeding change of country without slackening speed. The young of most marine animals achieve a perfect camouflage by the negation of all colour whatsoever, and not until they are old enough to make some show of self-defence do the larvæ of fishes, molluscs, and crustaceans, develop tell-tale spots of pigment, which, as they increase in size, finally spread over their entire bodies.

Camouflage in its most precise form—i.e., the ejection of smoke as practised in modern war—was in vogue with a number of animals countless years before man appeared on earth. Desert creatures "kick up a dust" when pursued, whilst certain marine animals, when disturbed or attacked, will shoot out a fluid from special glands with great effect both as regards covering a retreat and half blinding the enemy. The common cuttlefish secretes large quantities of a deep tinted "sepia" fluid, which is stored in a sac or "ink-bag" and is ejected with great force through the animal's syphon pipe whenever concealment by means of a "smoke screen" is desired. All the cephalopods produce this "sepia blind," but the sepia of commerce is obtained from the loligo or calamary, which is caught in great numbers off the shores of Southern Italy. The dried bags command about 35s. a pound. A large number of other molluscs enjoy the power of creating a smoke cloud. Many kinds of whelk can emit a voluminous screen, one species, *Murex brendaris*, having provided the Tyrian purple which was used by the ancients for their festal garments.

Several kinds of ground beetles, known as bombardier beetles, eject a volatile fluid when pursued. Upon coming into contact with the air the fluid vaporizes with a very audible explosion and with sufficient force to lay the pursuer, even if several times larger than the bombardier, upon its back. Finally, the skunk may be cited as a past-master in the art of camouflage as literally interpreted. The glandular secretion which emits the fearsome smell is, fortunately, used only sparingly, but the Zoo authorities have on several occasions been obliged to provide a keeper with a new suit of clothes—at short notice.

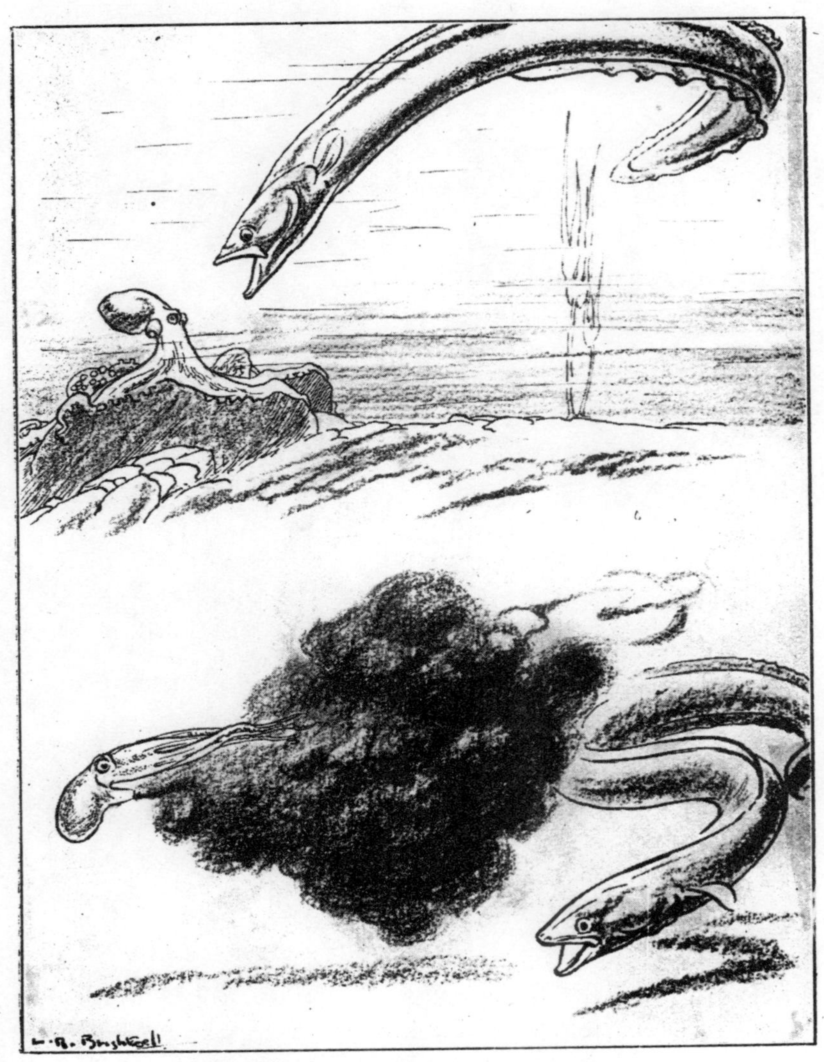

THE SMOKE-SCREEN (OCTOPUS *v.* CONGER).

[*p.* 160.

CHAPTER XIV

PLAGUES

THE so-called " Balance of Nature " is so delicately poised, and adjusted with such infinite nicety that the slightest touch may often throw it out of gear. Such a catastrophe may result in what is loosely known as a plague. Thus the indiscriminate persecution of the rat's natural foes, cats, weasels, polecats, and owls, may have a disastrous effect. The rash introduction of some animal or plant in a country foreign to it may likewise be the cause of misfortune. The Canadian water weed for instance has fairly choked certain parts of our fen country, whilst the introduction of rabbits into Australia and pigs into parts of New Zealand has, as is well known, brought with it the decimation of the native fauna. Many other examples can be cited to show the danger of thus interfering with Nature, and I propose to preface this chapter by quoting two specially noteworthy cases.

The representatives of a large island in the

Pacific Ocean who visited Europe many years ago where they saw goldfish for the first time, are no longer recipients of the plaudits of their countrymen. The beautiful golden fish exhibited in a public aquarium so impressed the dusky officials that there and then they decided to buy a large number and introduce them into their native ponds and rivers. This they proceeded to do with the result that the goldfish increased in such prodigious numbers that they actually exterminated the only edible fresh-water fish in the island. To add insult, so to speak, to injury, the goldfish soon ceased to be ornamental, reverting to their ancestral dirty grey-green coloration.

That the sea-lion like so many other creatures plays its part in the scheme of things is now fully appreciated by the former directors of a once highly successful guano company operating off the coast of California. The sea-birds that deposited the guano lived on fish which they shared with several large colonies of sea-lions. This fact eventually came to the notice of the members of the board, who passed sentence of death upon the sea-lions, thinking that if the latter were removed there would be more fish and as a natural sequence more guano. Rifles soon made short work of the unfortunate mammals, but from that day the birds that laid the golden manure departed for ever. The directors had not realized the fact that the swift-swimming and far-ranging sea-lions had acted as sheep dogs and rounded up the fish until they came within a few hundred yards of the coast and within striking distance of the birds. No sea-lions no fish, no fish—no birds, no birds—no guano, was the lesson learnt by the hard-headed but unimaginative business men.

But to revert to the subject of animal plagues: the most notable mammalian instance is that of the lemming, a rodent very abundant in many parts of Europe. At certain intervals enormous migrations of these creatures take place, trekking from all quarters until they meet to form a veritable river that destroys everything in its path. The depredations of foxes, hawks, owls, and man do little to stem the advance which usually terminates at the coast, where the animals perish.

That enemy of the human race, the rat, a creature responsible for so much damage to buildings, and disease, is not an indigenous animal, but invaded this country in the Middle Ages, having been brought on ships from the

Far East. To-day the damage for which this creature is annually responsible amounts to at least £25,000,000. Not a hundred years ago the inhabitants of Puffin Island off the coast of Wales were forced to abandon their holdings. Puffin Island is so called from the millions of puffins that made it their home along with a multitude of rabbits. No annoyance from rats had been experienced until the year 1817 when a German vessel was wrecked off the island. But after that, in consequence of the immigration of the animals from the wreck to the shore and their subsequent rapid increase in numbers, the rabbits and puffins were destroyed, and the island rendered uninhabitable was left in possession of the noxious rodents.

In many remoter parts of the country it used to be firmly believed that rats can be expelled by incantation. It is recorded that many years ago when the island of Lismore was invaded by rats the whole population joined in a rat-expelling song with the result that the animals left the island immediately, swimming in a solid mass across to the opposite mainland.

The following, quoted from Boelter's book *The Rat Problem*, is part of the successful rat-expelling incantation which has been translated from the Gaelic :

"A thousand ills befall thee, greedy rat!
Expertest thief that ever yet was born!
In barn and stackyard, maugre trap and cat,
Sad is the state of all my stock of corn;
Nor does a handful serve thee; shameless thief,
Unblushing rogue, thou claimest the whole sheaf!

Nor corn in sheaf, nor barley snugly stacked
Could serve thy turn; but all my garnered grain,
In well-filled sacks, is next by thee attacked.
And all is spoiled, thou thief of fertile brain;
And all my sacks are nibbled too, and holed—
A sight most aggravating to behold.

Alas! for all my seed corn in the spring!
Alas! for all thy keep, my good brown mare!
But take advice, and leave me, rat; and take
All thy companions with thee: else beware!
My malison shall fall withouten fail
On thee and thine, from whisker tip to tail.

So, rat, be warned, away! across the ferry,
And in some quarter else be sleek and merry;
By good St. Michael, and by chaste St. Bride,
I charge thee, leave me ere the morning tide!"

Many insect plagues have been the direct result of persecuting insect-eating birds. It is computed that in America at least seven hundred and fifty million pounds' worth of damage is done annually to crops by insect pests. In Ohio some years ago caterpillars held up the railways for five days, as their bodies, crushed in countless millions, rendered the metals so slippery that the wheels of the rolling stock refused to revolve upon them.

From very ancient times the plagues of locusts have been feared beyond all others.

It is of course related in the Bible how Jehovah in order to punish Pharaoh, who had not been behaving himself properly, commanded Moses to stretch forth his hand to make locusts spread over the whole of Egypt—"And Moses stretched forth his rod over the land of Egypt, and the Lord brought an east wind upon the land all that day and all that night; and when it was morning, the east wind brought the locusts. And the locusts went up over all the land of Egypt, and rested in all the coasts of Egypt; very grievous were they; before them were no such locusts as they, neither after them shall be such. For they covered the face of the whole earth, so that the land was darkened; and they did eat every herb of the land, and all the fruit of the trees which the hail had left; and there remained not any green thing in the trees, or in the herbs of the field through all the land of Egypt."

Pliny tells us that in Greece there was a law enforcing the inhabitants to wage war against the locusts three times in the year, during the periods when the eggs, larvæ, and adults were most abundant. In one of the islands of the Mediterranean the inhabitants were forced to pay as taxes so many measures of locusts. Figuier describes how the negroes of the Soudan endeavour to frighten the locusts in their flight by savage yells. In other countries the natives likewise attempt to intimidate the insects by firing a cannon. In the Middle Ages they exorcised the locusts, and the monk Alvarez has related how he employed exorcisms against a plague of these insects which he encountered in Africa. He made the natives form in procession and ordered them to chant sacred songs. "Thus chanting" he writes "we went into a country where the corn had been destroyed, and I made the natives catch a good many locusts to whom I delivered an adjuration which I carried with me in writing, admonishing and excommunicating them. Then I charged them in three hours' time to depart to the sea, or else go to the land of the Moors, leaving the land of the Christians. On their refusal I adjured and convoked all the birds of the air, animals, and tempests to dissipate, destroy, and devour them; for this admonition I had a number of locusts seized and having pronounced these words in their presence that they might not pretend to be ignorant of them, I let them go so that they might tell the rest." Figuier aptly remarks "if one reflects that on their arrival in the land of the Moors, these same locusts were probably received by prayers which had for their object the return of the locusts to the land of the Christians, the unfortunate insects must have been very much embarrassed by such contradictory adjurations."

We have advanced considerably since the days of Pharaoh, and now fight the locust hosts with such up-to-date gadgets as liquid fire, yet periodically the plague clouds still appear in Africa, India, Australia and even Southern Europe, darkening the sun, and covering every green thing with millions of hungry individuals that presently move on leaving nothing but the bare earth behind. Not only is the harvest devoured when the locust legions appear but the insects when finally beaten to the earth and reduced to mere mounds of rotting corpses may give rise to a train of pestilence as fatal to the farmer as was the living insect to his crops. The Arabs have aptly christened the locust the "licker up." From the moment when the infant locust emerges from the egg-shell, laid in the hard earth, he begins to eat. He is at first a wingless caricature of his parents and is then known by the name of "twister" from his rolling and rollicking mode of progression. Socn, however, he begins to hop and at the end of about twelve weeks the wings begin to bud and the creature moves forwards with a terrible steadfastness of purpose. A strange feature of the egg-laying is that the female is supported by two males whilst employing her ovipositor in the manner of a road-drill to ensconce her eggs in the ground.

In a correspondence in *Nature* some years ago a writer estimated that a great flight of locusts that he had witnessed crossing the Red Sea covered two thousand square miles of air and that the number of insects therefore exceeded twenty-four billions. He further calculated the weight of the total mass at 42,580 millions of tons, on the basis that each locust weighed one sixteenth of an ounce.

Scarcely less terrible, though fortunately of much rarer occurrence are the well organized advances of the driver ants of Equatorial Africa. Man and beasts, such as elephants and gorillas, must give way before them, abandoning lair or hut, not daring to dispute the path.

The little South American ant, though less terrible, is responsible for an enormous amount of damage not only in its native land but in various parts of the globe where it has been accidentally imported.

Of all the inhabitants of Madeira none are more unpopular than these ants, which were introduced into the island in samples of sugar cane less than forty years ago. The insects literally swarm everywhere up to a height of 3,000 feet, entering houses, and attacking everything edible. They have been responsible not only for the destruction of all the fruit trees, but have also entirely destroyed the coffee plantations, which before the advent of these undesirable aliens were a source of great profit to the inhabitants.

CHAPTER XV

LONGEVITY

A GIANT tortoise that was an intimate of the great Napoleon is still living on the island of St. Helena. Tortoises attain a greater age than any other animals, and, according to Lord Rothschild, an authority on these creatures, several examples in the Tring Museum weighing over 550 lb. must have been close on three centuries old when scientific claims put an end to their protracted existences. As the date when the St. Helena veteran was exiled from its native land of Aldabra is not recorded, and its age and size at the time are not known, the reptile, although probably the world's oldest inhabitant, is not in a position to lay any definite claim. The small European and North African land tortoises which are yearly imported to this country by the shipload, will, under proper conditions, live to a ripe, if not sensational, old age. One of these which died quite recently was for ninety-six years the pet of successive generations of a family in Cornwall. Only a few months before its death the animal on a very hot day pursued the gardener with such determination, biting at his trousers and butting at his feet, that it had to be shut up in the house. A land tortoise is stated to have belonged to the Bishops of Peterborough for about 220 years, whilst the shell of another ecclesiastical specimen, one acquired by Archbishop Laud in 1628, and which died 105 years later, is still exhibited to visitors at Lambeth Palace.

It is an established fact that the duration of life of the lower races of mankind is shorter than that of the more civilized. It will be learnt without surprise, therefore, that the average age attained by our poor relations the apes is not great, at least as judged from the human standpoint. Their potential longevity certainly does not exceed forty years. Micky, the chimpanzee who for a period held the proud position of "Father of the Zoo," lived for twenty-eight years in captivity, and was about three years old on his arrival at the Regent's Park menagerie, where he died of old age.

Although amongst mammals large animals as a rule live to a greater age than small ones, there is

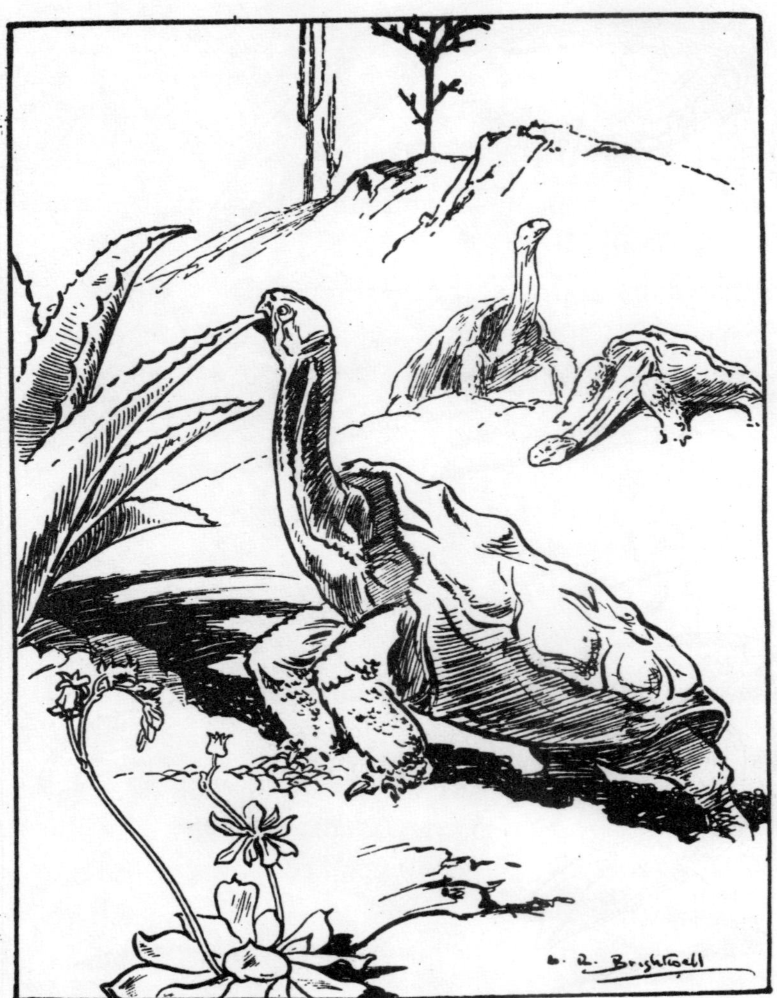

A VETERAN ABINGDON ISLAND TORTOISE

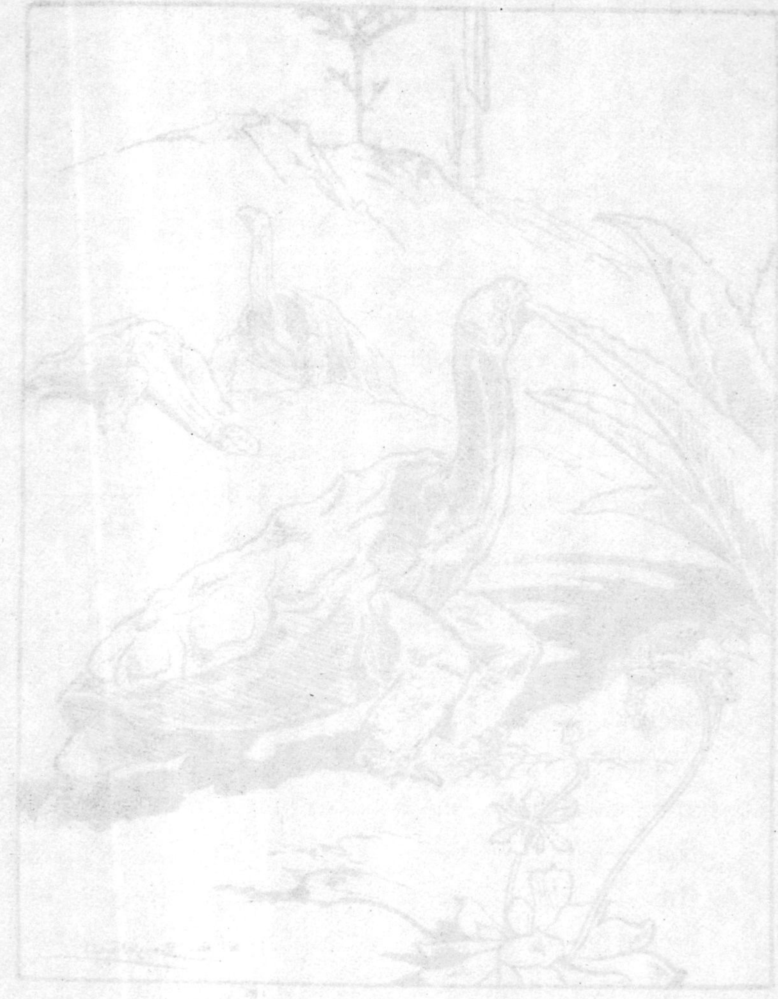

no constant relation between their size and potential longevity. Thus the maximum duration of life of a giraffe is less than that of a bat. Such gigantic animals as elephants and whales are credited with centuries of existence. They, however, reach their maximum size in a comparatively short period, and are often by no means as venerable as they appear. Jumbo, who measured eleven feet in height and weighed six and a half tons, attained his maximum development in twenty years. Elephants in proportion to their size have a low potential longevity, lower than that of man. There is, in fact, no authenticated record of an elephant of over seventy years. The official lists of the Indian Government, published some years ago, show that of 138 elephants only one lived for more than twenty years after it had been captured. It has been assumed that giant whales, which may reach a length of over 100 feet and a weight of eighty to ninety tons, are more than a century old Dr. Frederic A. Lucas, of the American Museum of Natural History, has recently completed a study of these monsters, and he finds that they reach their full size in comparatively few years. Our ideas as to their remarkable longevity must, therefore, undergo revision. The hippotamus and rhinoceros both flourish under captive conditions, and we are therefore able to give a fairly reliable indication of their potential longevity. In proportion to their size and weight they are short-lived. The once notorious "Guy Fawkes," a hippopotamus born in the Zoo in 1872, died of senile decay at the age of thirty-nine, whilst an Indian rhinoceros, which arrived at the Gardens when about two years old, likewise died of senility after only forty years of captivity.

The actual ages to which the mammals and birds in our Zoological Gardens have attained have been given by Dr. Chalmers Mitchell. The records of the carnivora support the view that they are fairly long-lived, bears having reached 33 years, lions and tigers 17, sea-lions 17, hyaenas and jackals 14, badgers 12, and foxes 10. Rodents, when we take their size into consideration, are to be regarded as living very long lives, the figures ranging from twenty years in the porcupine, fifteen in the squirrel, down to three in the dormouse. Many birds attain considerable ages. The following are some authenticated records: Egyptian vulture 118, golden eagle 104, parrot 102, swan 70, raven 69, eagle owl 68, herring gull 44, crane 43, pelican 41, peacock 40, dove 40, stork 36, ostrich 30, oyster-catcher 30, domestic fowl 30, cassowary 26, duck 26, nightingale 25, skylark 24, goldfinch 21, pheasant 21, canary 20, kiwi 20. The above figures show that in the birds as in the mammals there is no relation between longevity and size. Thus an ostrich can entertain no hope of attaining to half the age of a number of birds less than one-third its bulk.

Fish stories are notoriously untrustworthy. It is not surprising, therefore, to find that certain fish are credited with enormous spans of life. The voracious carp that appeal to the generosity of the public in the lake at Fontainebleau are reputed to be anything from two to three centuries old. The lake certainly harbours some enormous specimens, stated to be white with age. The fish are old, perhaps forty or even fifty years, but their "rime of age," is only to be attributed to a fungoid disease which coats them with a dense but unromantic frost. A French historian disposes of the fable of their antiquity by observing that in 1789, 1830, and 1848, the fish-ponds of Fontainebleau fell under the control of the sovereign people who loved the carp too well from a gastronomic point of view to permit size or age to be an obstacle to their ministering to their stomachs. The pike is another fish reputed to be very long-lived, but there is no proof that such is the case. The skeleton of a "pike" seventeen feet long and stated to be 267 years old was until recent years preserved at Mannheim. However, an examination of its bones by a specialist furnished proof of the fact that the giant had been manufactured out of a number of smaller fish.

Sturgeon and catfish live to a fair age. A number of fresh-water sturgeons living in Captain Vipan's private aquarium at Stibbingdon Hall were obtained from Russia over forty years ago, whilst a giant catfish from the Danube, which is at the present time an attraction at the Zoo Aquarium, is known to be well over fifty years old. The latter fish and another specimen of its kind still living in the lake at Woburn are the survivors of three imported by Lord Odo Russell in the year 1874. Another ancient inhabitant of the aquarium is the four-foot-long giant salamander of Japan, with a record dating back nearly forty years. The growth of this salamander, which was originally described as a fossil man, "Homo diluvii testis," has been studied by the writer. Young specimens put on an inch a year, but after attaining a length of two feet the rate of growth is considerably reduced, that of the forty-year-old specimen being less than one-eighth of an inch. As the creature has still more than a foot to grow before attaining to its maximum size, its potential duration of life is probably in the neighbourhood of 120 years, an age only exceeded by the members of the tortoise tribe.

Every year the Zoo authorities obtain an exact valuation of their charges which is required for the Zoological Society's annual accounts. This is not easily arrived at, for in valuing a wild animal it is necessary to have a knowledge not only of the creature's condition and age, but also of its average and potential length of life in captivity.

The Zoo curators find that the death-rate amongst new arrivals is rather heavy and that a number of animals take a few months to become acclimatized to their new conditions, after which they may live for many years. The "expectation of life" is higher after a few months of captivity than on arrival, and it therefore follows that the value of an animal is correspondingly greater or less in accordance with the time that has elapsed since its capture. Senility in certain wild animals is difficult to detect, and a knowledge of the potential longevity of the species is therefore required, as, although from the showman's point of view one that has lived in captivity for a certain number of months, or even years, is worth much more than a new arrival, there is, of course, a limit, and after a certain period its value decreases. Such are some of the facts that have to be taken into consideration by the Zoo curators in the course of their valuation.

The rhinoceros and the hippopotamus share the distinction of being the most valuable Zoo animals, each being worth close on £1,000. Giraffes when quite young are worth £500 or £600, but when old are unsaleable owing to the impossibility of transporting them—their necks being too high to pass through tunnels. Elephants are worth about £400 each and may earn £200 or £300 a year in carrying children. Apart from the popular favourites, a number of the animals which do not appeal to the visitor are of scientific value, and their deaths are anxiously awaited by the authorities of natural history museums and other zoological institutions.

The total value of the animals at present on exhibit in the Regent's Park menagerie is estimated at £30,000. This figure does not represent the full value cf the collection, but is merely an indication of what the Zoological Society would expect to receive from a forced sale of its animals —a circumstance which is, fortunately, never likely to arise.

CHAPTER XVI

TRAVELS AND MIGRATIONS

MIGRATION, that annual movement of animals from one place to another, has ceased to be the great mystery that it was once upon a time. Until late in the seventeenth century, however, the movements of birds were wholly wrapped in mystery, or explained in ways now discredited. The swallow, for instance, was commonly supposed to bury itself in the mud, and the early naturalists recounted how young fishermen, knowing no better, would often bring large hauls of swallows to land, each bound to its fellow by beak, toes and wings. The birds were placed in the sun to dry, where they presently took wing, and disported themselves until killed by the coming of the early winter night. The early Greeks and Romans interpreted the movements of the birds as best suited the religious or political atmosphere of the moment. Many Indian tribes, more practical in their way, have from early times made the birds their calendar, and named the months after those most prevalent at certain seasons.

Our present knowledge of bird migration is still very imperfect, but is built upon a firm rock of careful observation, carried on year after year at certain known stations. Valuable statistics have been compiled at lighthouses and special bird reservations and much has been learnt of bird travels by marking selected specimens with aluminium rings bearing a given address and date of marking. When a bird with such a passport attached falls into the hands of a person sufficiently interested to notify the sender, valuable knowledge concerning the creature's activities since the day of despatch is arrived at.

The steady increase of travel facilities is fast turning many of our own race into migrants. The first snap of winter sees the human of wealth and leisure in this country heading south beset with a mass of luggage, a batch of *visas* and other impedimenta. The swallow and many other birds hampered by no luggage make for the same direction. In the case of all migrants from our bleak shores, the reason for making the journey is the same—the desire for warmth. Some nomadic races have thus oscillated between hill and plain for countless centuries and a host of birds have done so ever since the first ice age. But the majority of birds are more fortunate than the humans since they know no dread of winter, being bred in this country during the early summer. They are prompted to move by a force which has been called "hereditary instinct," an instinct not always reliable and which at times leads to their downfall. Either they lose touch with older and more sophisticated individuals who have already made the journey, or by reason of their immaturity fail to survive the unexpected buffetings of chance. Young north-bound snipe have been driven to ground at Battersea, Wandsworth, Hammersmith, etc., whilst some years ago a woodcock was picked up one November day in Tothill Street near Westminster.

Many birds that appeal to the gourmet are trapped on their journeys. Thus the quail which winters in Africa, returning to Europe in the late spring, is captured in enormous numbers in Southern Europe. A headquarter of the quail harvest is the island of Capri where upon the first indication of the birds' arrival the entire island is ringed with nets in which the exhausted birds are captured and shot. Lighthouses situated on the route of migration are responsible for the deaths of millions of birds that blinded by the dazzling lights dash themselves to death against the glass or masonry.

"Homing Instinct" is a convenient term "coined" to describe these bird travels. With the carrier pigeon we are all familiar, but its achievements are easily eclipsed by many sea-birds. A few years ago exhaustive experiments were made with those inhabiting the Tartugas Islands in the Gulf of Mexico. Young terns were captured in the nesting season, marked and taken by ship eight hundred miles distant. They were well fed during transit but not allowed to "look out of the window." Twelve days after liberation the majority were home. The instinct of orientation in the common British toad is likewise very remarkable. Unlike the common frog which shows absolutely no discrimination in the choice of the locality in which it lays its eggs, the common toad chooses only special pools and ponds to breed in, making long journeys to reach them. On its way it may pass numerous sheets of water which to the common frog would appear eminently suitable for the purpose of laying. The travelling takes place by day as well as by night and should there happen to be a high road in the neighbourhood of the "rendezvous," hundreds of dead toads will be found run over by motor cars, the number of crushed corpses increasing in number as the proximity to the pond is approached. That the toads do not depend upon visual or hygroscopic cues to reach their breeding grounds can be proved by taking a number of individuals in a sack or basket from the selected pond to a considerable distance, and turning them loose—preferably near a locality where there is another pond. After a few preliminary hops all the toads will be observed to make a "bee line" in the direction of the sheet of water whence they were removed.

In spite of the fact that many theories have been suggested for explaining such feats, they still remain a mystery.

The animal travels recorded above are remarkable enough, but they are eclipsed by the journeys undertaken by the common eel. The eel is the possessor of a very small brain, yet annually billions fresh from their nurseries in mid-Atlantic make their way to Europe and not only ascend our English rivers, but penetrate the Scottish lochs, the Norwegian fjords, and even the Swiss lakes. This amazing journey is prefaced by an equally astonishing trip made first of all by the parents from their various European haunts to the common breeding ground -a distance of about three thousand miles—where the parents congregate and mate. The early stages of the egg laying and hatching are yet wrapped in mystery, but it is established that the young of the European eel make due East as soon as they are hatched. The journeys are begun in the early summer in deep water and in total darkness. Feeding on microscopic life they grow apace, and rise steadily in the water until caught in the moving currents about 100 feet from the surface. By the second summer nearly half the journey has been accomplished, and the immature eels have increased considerably in length. At this period they are quite transparent, and leaf-shaped. Immature eels were not known to scientists before the middle of the past century, for although carefully examined and made the subject of much controversy they were not known to be eels. It was not until 1890 that their place in the scheme of things was definitely located.

Ever moving Eastwards, in their third summer the creatures are within European waters. With the coming of the autumn they change shape, losing their resemblance to a leaf and become cylindrical. At this stage, when little thicker than a needle, they eat nothing. Their teeth have dropped out, their eyes are formed, and a tiny red blob marks the situation of the heart. They are now known as elvers, and in this form enter our big tidal rivers in shoals of many million strong. Up to quite recently the little fish were caught in great numbers and made into eel puddings, a pound of eel pudding containing over two thousand elvers. Of course during the journey across the Atlantic the ranks of these vast shoals are thinned considerably. Fish and sea birds of all kinds take toll of them, as do innumerable crabs and jellyfish. Vast numbers are smothered in great masses of the floating ascidian "salpa."

"Eel fares" which once marked the arrival of young eels in tidal waters are now almost extinct. For the most part the young eels are permitted to ascend the streams in peace, and to grow and fatten in the upper reaches. But the eel is a born traveller and is always ready for a change of scene. Its appetite is enormous, and when the food supply in a given locality shows signs of exhaustion it prospects for a less over-fished locality. Through its capacity for living out of water for a protracted period it makes long overland journeys, and few sheets of water are closed to it. For instance, elvers do not ascend the Danube, and yet eels occur in that river, into which they gain admittance via canals, ditches and tributaries of the Rhine. Eels are found in almost any large irrigation system in isolated ponds, reservoirs, swimming baths, and even in the Swiss lakes 3,000 feet above sea level. A demonstration of the eel's lust for adventure was given recently at the Zoo, where a specimen persisted night after night in climbing out of the aquarium allotted to it and visiting one several tanks away inhabited by a collection of sea anemones. Its determination to choose its own quarters was such that the aquarium officials eventually had to give in to it.

When the eel reaches maturity at the age of five or six, having attained a length of three feet or more, it commences the return journey to where it came from. It travels fasting, and, although whilst still in fresh-water too big to fear many of the foes which menaced it on its journey eastward, has now to run the gauntlet of its deadliest enemy—man. It is now a marketable fish and lines, nets, and dozens of other devices threaten it on its journey seawards. Once in open water, sea birds, sharks, porpoises, and other creatures work havoc amongst the homing eels. Sufficient, however, return to the place of their birth to lay the eggs which will eventually start another eel-invasion heading across the Atlantic.

The salmon's "wanderlust" has been known for many years, and is better understood than that of the eel. When about three years old, and having assumed a silvery livery, the salmon leaves the river in which it was born, and makes for the sea where it feeds and sports in gay bachelor or spinsterhood until Nature calls upon it to fulfil its destiny and ensure the continuance of the race. Then it ascends the river and, as recent research has proved, almost invariably the river of its birth. Frank Buckland has given an account illustrating the homing instinct of this fish. A friend of his who owned an island on the west coast of Scotland, netted a pool and out of the salmon caught carefully marked a number of specimens. He then put these fish in a tank on board his yacht, sailed right round his island, and then up a creek to the mouth of a river in which the salmon were liberated. This river although close to the river in which they were caught was in no way connected with it having a different watershed. It was as though the salmon had been carried from one base of an enormous horseshoe round to the other base. Most of these marked fish were caught during the same season in the neighbourhood of the pool in which they were originally caught up. The fish had returned to the river of their birth, a circuit of over forty miles from the locality where they were turned out and they must have passed six or seven tributaries up which they did not ascend although there was nothing to prevent their doing so. In its progress towards the upper reaches the salmon contends with all kinds of obstacles, battling with powerful rapids and leaping waterfalls often ten feet high. Naturally the weaker fish fall by the wayside. To ensure the safe arrival of more fish at the breeding grounds the salmon ladder has been evolved on many reaches. This consists of a number of huge wooden or concrete troughs arranged in ascending series thus breaking up an impossible 25-foot jump into a number of moderate leaps which any healthy fish can easily negotiate.

The movements of sea fish are very strange and our many marine biological stations with their elaborately equipped trawlers and survey ships are likely to be engaged on the subject for many years to come. The mystery of the life history of the sea lamprey has in recent years been elucidated. It ascends rivers to spawn just as does the salmon. Unlike the salmon, however, it does not return to the sea alive and well to repeat the journey, but dies on the return, worn out with its labours of building a nest upon some submerged gravel bed. After the breeding season the lampreys are literally "worn to rags," their skins frequently being in ribbons.

Many fish travels are not necessarily connected with courtship. The vast exodus of herring from Norwegian shores to the Channel every autumn is probably a matter of changing feeding grounds, and the annual influx of porpoises and seals is the natural outcome of those animals following the shoals of fish which in their turn are pursuing organisms that change their grounds according to seasonal variations in the temperature of the water. Food is in fact at the bottom of those animal journeys—where there is not a lady in the case.

A wonderful instance of travelling *en masse* is furnished by the fur seal. At the clarion call of spring the seals of the Northern Pacific suddenly renounce their care-free sports and feasting for a two thousand mile trek, often through tempestuous seas, to the St. Paul's Rocks and certain other more Southern localities, where, protected by game laws and largely hidden to view in the ever recurrent fogs, they fight, woo and bring forth their families. For weeks on end they neither eat nor drink and there can be little opportunity for sleep. The males about five times as bulky as the females arrive some weeks in advance of the brides to be.

Amongst reptiles the turtle offers a good example of a creature that will make little of mere distance if there is the perpetuation of the race to be ensured at the journey's end. Turtles are entirely aquatic, but once a year the pregnant females journey shorewards to lay their eggs. Once arrived at their destination they struggle painfully inland until they are well beyond the range of high tide when they lay their eggs beneath the sand.

The migrations of the larvæ of an insect (Sciara) are amongst the most mysterious of all phenomena. The creatures which have no feet are found in immense trains formed by the union of a sticky secretion. The collections composed of thousands of these creatures clinging to each other resemble an elongated serpent. They advance with one accord in a certain direction and if on their journey they encounter stone or log they either turn round it, or else divide into two sections, which join up again after the obstacle has been passed. In the event of a column being divided, the two parts quickly reunite, the hindmost portion hurrying for all it is worth to catch up with the one in front. If the posterior part of this assembly be joined up with the anterior, a circle is formed which may keep on revolving for several hours before breaking up.

Guérin-Méneville states that these larvæ which normally live in the ground are occasionally obliged to come to the surface in order to seek at a distance a place where they will find suitable food or an appropriate locality to undergo their metamorphosis. He is of opinion that the uniting of these thousands of individuals can be best explained by the necessity for mutual protection against drying up after leaving the ground, the creatures deriving moisture by the glutinous matter which connects them.

Some other journeyings of insects and their larvæ have been referred to in a previous chapter. Quite as mysterious as any swarming of ants or locusts are the periodic movements of certain land crabs. The giant "coco-nut crab" or robber crab of Christmas Island, which has been observed to climb lofty trees, makes a frequent peregrination to the coast to moisten its gills, and these journeys are fraught with danger. The robber crab has a mass of fat under its tail which appeals strongly to many animals, including man. Pitched battles

THE ROBBER OR COCO-NUT CRAB.

[p. 194.

often take place between these crabs and rats, the latter despite their superior brains and agility not always coming off victorious. The robber crab's body may measure over a foot in length. The creature is endowed with very great strength and Darwin has related how specimens placed in large biscuit tins secured by wire, have escaped by punching holes through the tin. Matrimonially intent, land-crabs of all tropical countries make annual pilgrimages to the sea. On a certain spring day the entire land-crab population, which may amount to several millions of crabs, issues forth and the procession headed by the males may be several miles long and forty to fifty feet wide. No obstacle however great will turn them from their path. In the course of the journey houses are frequently invaded and the onward progress of the creatures has been described as scarcely less terrifying than that of the redoubtable driver ants of Central Africa.

CHAPTER XVII

TEETH

MAN, as the old saying truly said, is fearfully and wonderfully made, and his teeth are not amongst the least vital or wonderful of his possessions, since their efficiency or otherwise largely dictates the policy of his other organs. Teeth, in fact, may be the real masters of our fates. Passing the teeth of man in review one fact stands out, namely, that those of the more primitive races show a marked superiority over those of the average inhabitants of our great cities. The human mouth is from a dental point of view one of the strangest collections of anomalous forms ever gathered together in so small a space. Where the wild animal has, according to its kind, specialized, man has generalized, with result that each kind of tooth has become reduced in size and form from Nature's original standards. Man uses his incisors only for nibbling soft food, whilst his canines are almost entirely unemployed. Apes and monkeys, however, use these same teeth not only for cracking bones and nuts, but for fighting, the canines of baboons rivalling those of the largest carnivora and being used for the same purpose—attack. In fact in many extinct cats these teeth were developed to such an extent that they resembled the tusks of the walrus. These overgrown teeth often had saw-like edges, and reached their maximum development in the sabre-toothed tiger.

Great canine teeth are generally associated with beasts of prey, but they can be used for aggression by most animals. Several kinds of deer, such as the muntjac, musk deer, and chevrotain have theirs developed into tusks, giving the wearers a very pugnacious appearance. The huge tusks of the walrus are simply canine teeth which have become exaggerated by constant exercise in the peaceful pursuit of digging clams out of the mud, or helping their possessor to hook himself on to the edge of ice floes. They are also used for fighting and, as revealed in a recent film, to awaken sleeping comrades upon the approach of danger, when all lurch from the floating ice into the safety of the sea.

There are instances in which a single series of teeth may dominate the entire animal. Thus in the Arctic Narwhal, the incisors are virtually the only functioning teeth and have in the male developed into tusks from three to five feet in length. Where two are developed both twist spirally in the same direction, in marked contrast to the spiral horns of other animals where one always twists to the right, the other to the left. These tusks are apparently used for fighting purposes only—the narwhal's prey consisting almost entirely of squids which are swallowed whole.

The elephants, and the great army of rodents have become world famous through their incisor teeth. The well-known tusks of the former have been developed during long ages of constant usage from teeth little larger than those of a pig. Some of the earliest elephants had two pairs of tusks in each jaw, and each pair had cutting edges which worked one upon the other. As time progressed, however, the elephant relied more and more solely upon the upper tusks, with the result that the lower dwindled to insignificance, and finally disappeared. A few elephants used the lower tusks at the expense of the upper which atrophied. These forms are not wholly extinct, whereas at least two species that persisted in using only the upper tusks, still exist—on sufferance. The elephant's tusks, invaluable for up-

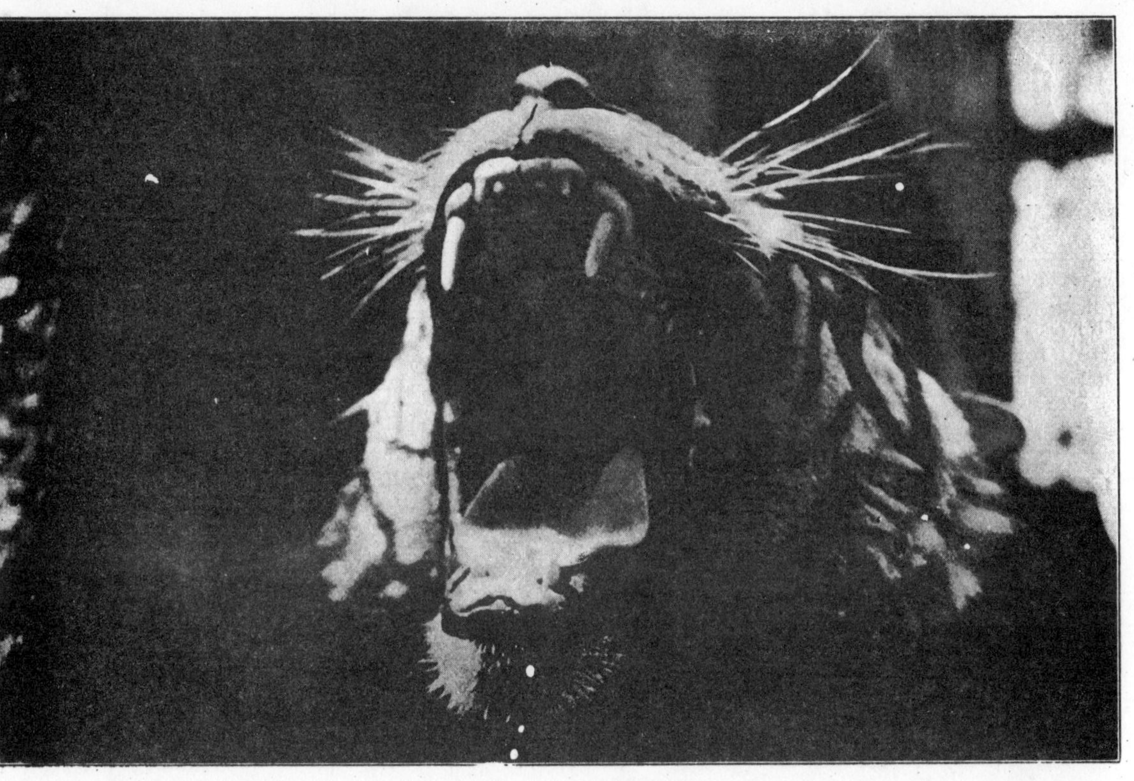

THE TIGER SHOWS HIS TEETH. [p. 198.

rooting trees, repulsing attack, or bullying, have been the creature's undoing, and but for Government intervention, the elephants of Africa and India would long since have disappeared. The ivory trade has in the past been the cause of wholesale slaughter and considerable feud and bloodshed between man and man.

Overgrown incisors may be a source of trouble in a variety of ways. At the beginning of the past century a large Indian elephant was brought to England, and by his exemplary behaviour became an almost national hero. He was exhibited at various shows and performed in the Drury Lane pantomime. His headquarters was Pidcock's menagerie at " Exeter Change," –a large building in the Strand. In 1826 tooth trouble set in and one night mad with toothache the giant animal ran amok in the building, crowded with other wild beasts and spectators. A terrible scene ensued until a squad of infantry was hurried to the spot and discharged over a hundred bullets into the unfortunate animal. The skeleton, riddled with bullet holes now stands in the College of Surgeons' Museum.

In 1850, the enterprising Frank Buckland was more successful with a big " hippo " also driven to frenzy by the decayed root of an upper incisor.

A keeper for whom the animal had a special aversion was employed to decoy it to the bars, when it was roped and chained. The operator then went into action with a two-foot pair of forceps, and the offending ivory was extracted.

With their chisel teeth, which can only be kept to a convenient length by a constant use, rats do many thousands of pounds' worth of damage, attacking with disastrous effect such varied substances as cement, oak, iron and lead. These incisor teeth reach a maximum development in the Beaver, their roots measuring six times the length of the exposed enamelled portion. An adult beaver can fell a tree three feet in circumference in eighteen hours, and should in the process one or both of these teeth be broken the stump continues to grow. But owing to the destruction of its cutting edge it cannot be kept in check by constant gnawing; with the result that it grows and grows, curving upwards and forwards in a circular route. In time it may pass over the top of its owner's head, rendering feeding impossible, and old specimens not infrequently thus meet a lingering death by starvation.

Amongst pigs the canines turn upwards and by growing continually form almost circular structures with their points resting on the animal's cheeks. In the Babirussa Pig of the Celebes, the upper tusks arrive at such excessive development that they serve their pugnacious owner as a sort of fencing mask.

In purely carnivorous animals the back teeth—the pre-molars, molars or grinders are more or less knife-edged, whilst in the seal they are finely fluted, a special provision for straining off the scales from living fish sucked in hastily below water. Where a vegetarian diet is the rule the back teeth become squat and massive, with their upper surfaces broken up into a series of complicated folds.

Teeth are out of fashion with modern birds, but there is evidence that they were once largely worn especially by the fish-eating divers. The teeth were set loosely in the jaw like those of many modern lizards, but as time progressed their place was taken by deep serrations of the horny sheath enclosing the upper and lower mandibles.

Most teeth are capable of inflicting a bite which is liable to turn septic, but certain animals have developed teeth that as conveyers of poison outshine the vilest efforts of the Borgias. With the single exception of the Helóderm Lizard of the desert regions of Arizona all the venomous reptiles are snakes. They have some of the upper teeth provided with grooves or channels connected with poison glands. When in action the fangs are exposed and the head raised until they are horizontal; then at lightning speed they are launched at the foe or prey and driven into the flesh. At the same time the glands are compressed and a jet of poison squeezed down each fang into the wound. The fangs are literally hypodermic syringes and are continually being replaced as they become worn out or broken.

Primarily such weapons are used to secure and paralyse the prey, the poison being innocuous to the snake secreting it; it is indeed regarded by many as a development of the digestive juices. Unfortunately the teeth do not always come into play only at meal times. It is computed that in India alone 25,000 persons annually meet their deaths at the fangs of the cobra, krait and Russel's viper. The preparation of anti-venomous toxins is now a cult in most civilized countries, but most snake charmers practise a rough and ready sort of inoculation, allowing themselves to be bitten slightly by young snakes at regular intervals, or deliberately operating upon themselves with the extracted poison.

The teeth of fishes, the lowest of the vertebrates, have much in common with those of reptiles, and like the snakes' teeth are used mostly for holding. They slope backwards toward the gullet, belonging to the "entrance, no exit" type. Often they interlock, and do so in certain deep sea forms on the outside of the fish's head.

The earliest fish had virtually no teeth at all, relying no doubt upon suctorial lips fringed with serrations like the modern lamprey. With the appearance of the sharks the tooth came into its own. One primeval shark had about four hundred fang-like teeth with cutting edges. To thoroughly appreciate the powers of the shark's tooth it is necessary to have been a spectator of the "haul up" on a Western Ocean trawler. Certain parts of the Atlantic swarm with blue sharks, and as soon as a net full of fish is drawn to the surface they appear in scores with the suddenness of a flock of vultures. Despite the efforts of the crew they often succeed in tearing the net to ribbons in a few minutes and cutting yard-long pieces of fish into pieces, as though armed with gigantic shears.

The teeth possessed by the six-inch long Cariba fish of the Amazon waters may be the undoing of the jaguar or even man himself. The fish congregate in vast shoals and should a large animal such as a tapir enter the water to drink, or essay to ford the stream in their vicinity, the creature is immediately surrounded and literally made mince-meat of by its diminutive foes.

Even more to be dreaded than the shark or the cariba is the Barracuda, a large fish inhabiting the warmer waters of various countries. Its teeth are set in sockets and only cast iron is immune to them. These large mullet-like fish have been frequently known to bite off the paddle of a canoe, and in Florida they are responsible for many bathing fatalities.

The fish having the most dangerous dentition in British waters is undoubtedly the large wolf fish, a giant blenny abounding in all waters north of Flamborough Head and south of Greenland. Fishmongers sell it under the aristocratic name of "rock salmon," but in Iceland it is known as the wolf fish or "stone breaker." With its dog-like front teeth it can snap a broom handle and make appreciable dents in a steel wire rope. Its throat and palate are furnished with pavement-like teeth that can crack the hardest cockleshells, and reduce a lobster to pulp.

Even coral rock is not safe from the File Fish of the West Indies, the fish habitually chiselling off lumps for the sake of the minute animals it contains. Molluscan teeth show a very remarkable arrangement, especially in the case of the whelks. Their teeth which vary much in size and shape are arranged in a row upon a long ribbon-like tongue which can lick its way through an inch-thick oyster shell. They act in the manner of a file, and though many come to grief in tackling hard substances, others are ever ready to fill up the ranks, and carry on the work of destruction.

CHAPTER XVIII

THE TAIL-PIECE

MAN and his near relatives, the man-like apes, have forced their tails to take a back seat as a result of their habit of persistently sitting upon them. A few other animals have little use for the caudal appendage, and in reviewing animals' tails we may find this organ in every stage of atrophy. A few domestic creatures have lost theirs as a result of intensive breeding and selection, but the almost tailless condition of such wild beasts as the bears and hippos is to be accounted for by the fact that their primitive ancestors when provided with tails neglected to make any use of them.

But as a rule the tail is well in evidence, having been put to a bewildering variety of uses. It may serve as a hand, a weapon, a tool, a seat, a blanket, a fly-whisk, or merely an ornament. The long pole used by the slack-wire walker is indispensable to his maintaining his equilibrium. Watch a rat running up a hawser or a long-tailed cat such as the leopard making its way along a branch, and it will be seen that the tail moves from side to side just as does the long pole carried by the music-hall tight-rope artist. It is equally valuable as a counterpoise on the ground, when the animal progresses on its hind legs only. But for their long tails such creatures as the jerboa and wallaby would fall forwards on their noses when travelling at high speed. In the living Frilled Lizards, as was the case with their ancestors the extinct bird-footed Dinosaurs, the tail serves materially in helping the animal to maintain the upright pose. Exertion eventually calls for a rest, and again the tail proves itself a friend in need. In nearly all the bipedal mammals the tail serves wholly or partially to support the body when at rest. The Jerboas and Gerbils curve theirs in the form of an S and place the tip only upon the ground. In the case of the Kangaroos, however, four-fifths of the appendage rests firmly on the ground, the animals sitting back upon it, as one would upon a shooting stick. There is abundant evidence that the Giant Sloths of Patagonia sat back upon their enormous tails and pelvic bones, and thus mounted upon a huge tripod grappled with lofty trees and despoiled them of their foliage.

The King Penguin is one of the few birds possessing a "shooting seat" tail, and it is a quaint sight to see the creature sitting well back with the toes elevated skywards at an angle of forty-five degrees. A very massive tail is possessed by the beaver. It is a good deal more than just a seat, serving as a very efficient rudder. It is not as old-time naturalists declared also used as a trowel, but is employed as an alarm gun. The beaver concentrates upon his job to the exclusion of all outside distractions, and a "gang" when at work on dam or lodge might easily be surprised by an enemy, but for the timely warning of the sentinel. One resounding smack of the tail upon the stream surface and he and his mates vanish precipitately until the "All clear" is given. The "warning tail" takes many strange forms. The rabbit offers a classic example, and its white "bob" seen travelling at high speed acts as a warning to all other rabbits in the neighbourhood to do likewise. The deer's tail is framed in a horse-shoe shaped frame of dark hair and serves the same purpose.

The Giant Ant-Eater of South America is the possessor of a luxuriant fan-shaped tail, and by

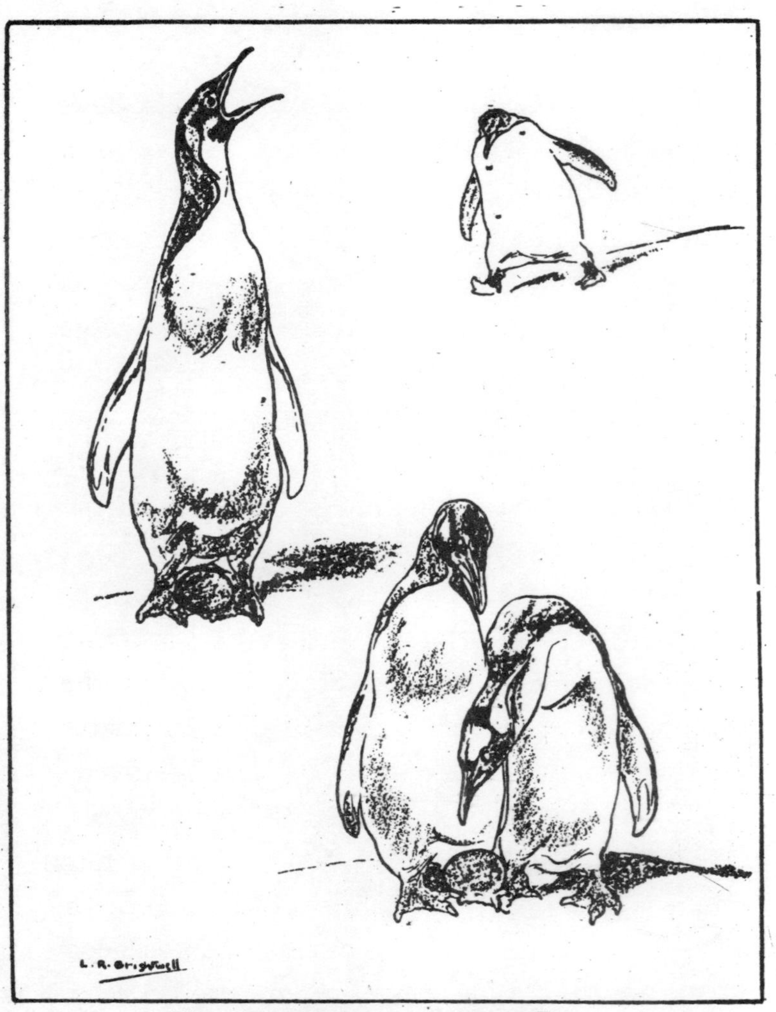

KING PENGUINS INCUBATING THEIR EGGS

holding it above its head and back makes it do duty for a sunshade.

When the hair is confined to the tip, the organ serves as a fly-whisk. Such whisks are of great length in the Giraffe and many kinds of antelope and are frequently annexed by man to perform the same useful office for himself.

The prehensile tail which doubtless took many millions of years to evolve is employed by a number of arboreal animals. In the spider monkeys the long tails are used as grasping organs enabling them to hang from the branches of trees without the help of their limbs. In some forms the tail is used as a " fifth hand " and at the Zoo some of these entertaining creatures may be observed accepting edible gifts and transferring them to their mouths by means of their highly specialized caudal appendages.

The Tree Ant-Eaters of Brazil employ their tails to swing from branch to branch when foraging for wasps' nests. The bear-like Kinkajou from the forest regions of Guiana has an unusually long tail which is used for climbing and grasping, and Zoo visitors enjoy seeing the animal, after hanging from the roof of its cage in an inverted position, deliberately climb back hand over hand up its own caudal appendage. The tree porcupines have powerful "hand tails," and one member of the cat family, the Binturong, is similarly provided. In nearly all cases the prehensile tail is well developed at birth. This is strikingly evident in the Australian and American Opossums where the newly-born young—about half a dozen in number—literally "strap hang" whilst riding on the parental back, each infant securely twisting its tail round that of the mother.

The possibility of making use of the caudal extremity as a weapon was realized by the first lizards. Often the tail was armed with spines over two feet in length and must have constituted a flail against which few rivals could hope to keep their feet. In modern lizards the tail is still the principal weapon. Those that have not their tails heavily armoured like the Australian Moloch, the Mexican Horned Lizard, the Egyptian Mastigures, the South African Zonures, can throw off the organ at a moment's notice and whilst the would-be captor occupies himself with the gyrating fragment, make good their escape. The big monitor lizards or "dragons" can use the tail with great effect and several Zoo keepers have received painful slashes over their calves and ankles. The crocodile's tail is capable of smashing a native canoe, hurling its crew into the water.

The emotion with which the whole animal is charged often oozes out of the tip of the tail, expressing anger, impatience, anxiety or joy. The importance of the organ under review as an index to a dog's character was thus quaintly expressed in an army form upon the breeds most useful for scouting, guard and ambulance duties : " . . . the tail carried erect, or curved sideways over the back, denotes a levity of character ill suited to military requirements."

It is probable that the first use to which the tail was put was simply that of propulsion. It is used thus amongst most primitive animals, and almost universally to this day amongst fishes. In the sting-ray it is, however, principally a weapon, the motor power being supplied by the immense pectoral fins. In the thresher shark it is developed into a sickle-shaped flail, whilst in the sea-horse it is as much a " hand " as is that of the spider monkey. Amongst birds the tail proper would seem to be solely to support the feathers—except in such rare instances as the penguin, where as previously mentioned it may be utilized as a seat. As a support to feathers it constitutes a most important item of adornment, and like some of the elaborately crested lizard tails and luxuriant mammalian appendages goes far to win for its owner much coveted approval in the mating season.

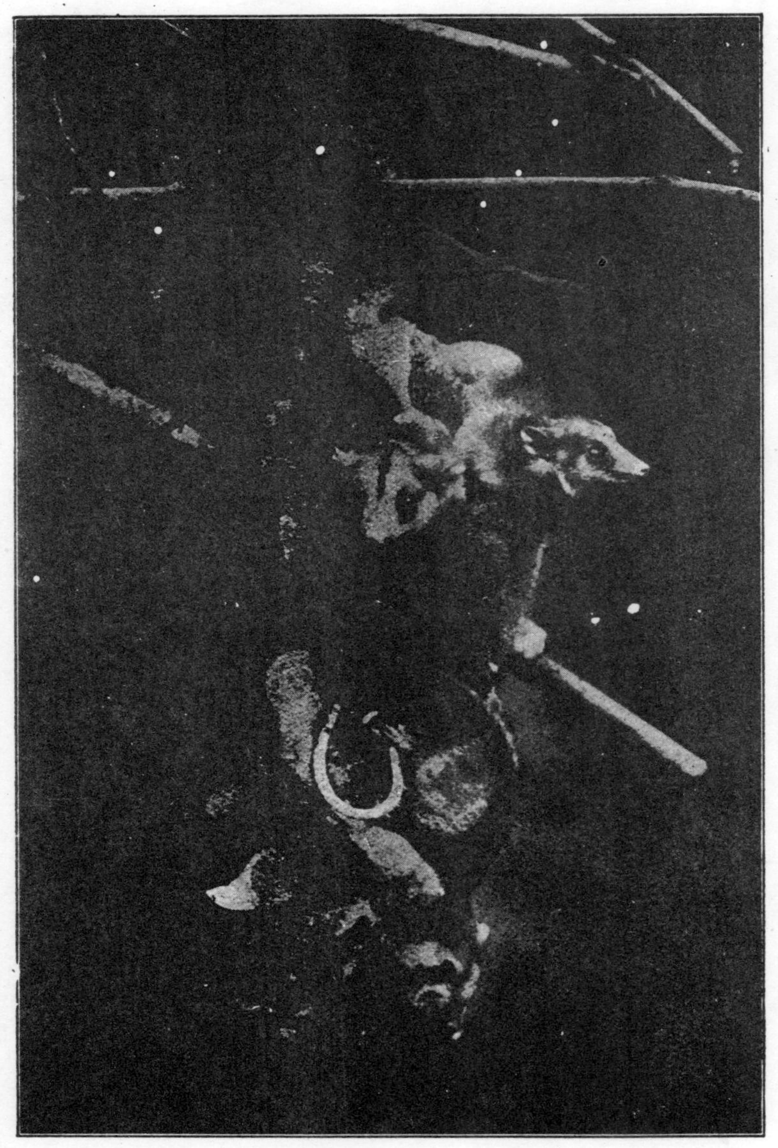

"STRAP-HANGING" OPOSSUMS.

[p. 212.